Diabetes is not a piece of cake®

> ## Prescribed for family, friends, & co-workers of folks with diabetes

Revised Fourth Edition

by Janet Meirelles, R.N., B.S.N.
Certified Diabetes Educator
Certified Health Education Specialist
Past Member Editorial Board, *Diabetes Forecast*

Foreword by: Andrew J. Ahmann, M.D.
Illustrated by: Lee Wright

Lincoln Publishing Incorporated
Lake Oswego, Oregon

Lincoln Publishing Incorporated
http://www.800books4u.com
Tel: (503) 699-1000
Post Office Box 1499
Lake Oswego, OR 97035-0499
U.S.A.

This book is not intended as a substitute for medical advice of physicians. The reader should
regularly consult a physician in matters relating to his or her health and particularly with respect
to any symptoms and/or concerns that may require diagnosis or medical attention.

Publisher's Cataloging-in-Publication Data

    Meirelles, Janet.
        Diabetes is not a piece of cake :
        prescribed for family, friends, and co-workers of folks with diabetes / author,
        Janet Meirelles ; foreword by, Andrew J. Ahmann ; illustrated by, Lee
        Wright. — Lake Oswego, OR: Lincoln Pub. Inc., c1994, 1995, 1997, 2010.

    P. : ill. ; cm.

    Includes bibliographical references, glossary, and index.

    ISBN: 978-1-884929-09-0

    1. Diabetes—Popular works.   2. Diabetes.
I. Title

    RC660.4M   616.462 dc20
                    2009939559

Revised Fourth Edition
ISBN 978-1-884929-09-0
Library of Congress Catalogue Number 2009939559

Trademarks: All brand names and product names used in this book are trademarks,
registered trademarks, service marks, or trade names of their respective holders.
Neither the publisher not the author has received any compensation from any vendor
of any product mentioned herein.

Printed in the United States of America

Foreword

by ANDREW J. AHMANN, M.D.

Diabetes is not a piece of cake ... fills a real void in what's available for the family, friends, colleagues and classmates of people with diabetes. In it you will find out what to do and what to avoid doing to help the person you care about who has diabetes. Subjects discussed vary from social situations to emergencies. From appropriate recipes and going to restaurants, to the symptoms of low and high blood glucose levels, and what you can do.

There are easy to understand and thoughtful explanations of the disease, which will give you an insight into what's happening– you won't merely get dry meaningless instructions.

Even if you have diabetes, and haven't kept up with the latest research, or if you've been too embarrassed to ask questions, there's important information in this book for you too.

There's a thorough glossary, a good index, a supplemental reading list and a summary of resources.

The author also corresponded with, received and reviewed hundreds of questionnaires from people who have diabetes and their family members and shares the insights she gained.

Since your chances of getting diabetes increase with aging, you'll find practical hints on what can be done to reduce those chances–AND, you'll discover reasons that may motivate you to take action now!

This well researched book is pleasant to read, thorough, thoughtful and includes the most recent developments. I hope you will find the time to read it.

Dr. AHMANN, in addition to his private practice as an endocrinology specialist, is Director of Harold Schnitzer Diabetes Health Center; and Professor of Medicine, Division of Endocrinology, Diabetes, and Clinical Nutrition at Oregon Health Sciences University. Dr. Ahmann is Past President of the American Diabetes Association, Oregon Affiliate. Dr. Ahmann has received many academic honors, awards, fellowships, and scholarships.

Acknowledgments

My heartfelt thanks to my husband Tom who encouraged me to write this book and helped in a hundred ways to see it through to its completion.

Special thanks to Andrew Ahmann, M.D. for his encouragement and Foreword; to the late James Hansen, M.D., formerly Medical Director of Emanuel Children's Diabetes Center for his insight into the special challenges of treating children with diabetes, to Michael Fulop, Psy.D. for his psychological expertise on children and adolescents with diabetes, and to Donald Adams, D.D.S., M.S., Past President of the American Academy of Periodontology and Professor and Chair Emeritus of Oregon Health Sciences University Department of Periodontology.

A special thank you to Bev Bromfield, Program Director of the Oregon and SW Washington American Diabetes Association affiliate for her untiring dedication to facilitating programs that educate people with diabetes and their families.

And I'm grateful to Lee Wright for his illustrations that humorously show some of the attitudes and pitfalls of having diabetes.

Many thanks also to my colleagues of the Oregon Diabetes Educators who made valuable suggestions. In particular, I wish to thank Patricia Maddix, RD; Jill Rose, RN; Nancy Autio, RN; Jody Babson, Sandra Birchall-Jones, RN; Diana Hayes, RN; Martha Hirsch, RD; Carol Schrader, RD; and Marge Thompson; RN.

And thanks to the hundreds of pen pals from Saudi Arabia to Washington who answered my questions, educated me, and told me how much they wanted to share their challenge.

iv

About the Author

Janet Meirelles is a Registered Nurse, a Certified Diabetes Educator and Certified Health Education Specialist. In recent years she has specialized in matters related to diabetes care. She has surveyed hundreds of people who have diabetes and discussed with them their important issues. These issues and experiences led her to write this book about what non-diabetics out to know and how they can help.

For several years Ms. Meirelles was in charge of a California and Los Angeles County sponsored supplemental services program, an important goal of which was the education about and self-management of diabetes by those within the program. The program she ran received honors and recognition.

Ms. Meirelles is a former member of the Editorial Board of the American Diabetes Association magazine, *Diabetes Forecast,* and has been published therein.

Ms. Meirelles is licensed to practice in Oregon, Washington, and California. She graduated from UCLA with a Bachelor of Science in Nursing and from the University of New Mexico with a Bachelor of Arts in Anthropology. Both degrees were awarded with academic honors.

Ms. Meirelles is now in private practice as a diabetes educator, an Adjunct Professor at the Institute for Health Care Professionals, and a diabetes support group facilitator in the Portland, Oregon area. She travels nationally giving talks about diabetes to lay and professional audiences.

Contents

Foreword iii

1   Not Everyone with Diabetes Is the Same 9

2   The History of Diabetes 16

3   What Does Diabetes Do? 23

4   Treatments–Different Pokes for Different Folks 34

5   So Many Chores, So Little Time 56

6   The Diabetes Diet–More Than Just No Sugar 75

7   Inviting Someone With Diabetes
    to Your Home for a Meal .101

8   Dining Out With Someone With Diabetes 119

9   Low Blood Sugar: When Sugar Is Medicine 135

10 High Blood Sugar: From Flu to ICU 154

11 Complications Go from Head to Toe 162

12 Exercise: The Good, the bad, and the ugly 184

13 Sex, Love, and Diabetes: Not Just Hormones 209

14 Pregnancy: A Labor of Love 224

15 Diabetes Is Tougher When You're a Kid 230

16 Feelings: Everybody Has Them 244

17 Diabetes–A Pain in the Wallet 263

18 Do I Have It? Will I Get It? 270

Appendix - Recipes 276

Appendix - Resources 298

Glossary 301

Index 314

1

Not Everyone With Diabetes is the Same

Why do some people with diabetes:

> take injections?
> take pills instead of injections?
>
> eat candy?
> not eat candy?
>
> test their blood sugar?
> not test their blood sugar?
>
> become blind or suffer other complications?
> not get any complications?

The answers are in this book. Plus, we'll discuss what you can do to help your co-worker, friend, or family member with diabetes.

First, I'd like to introduce you to two people I know with diabetes. They're very different but they also have some things in common.

Pat's Story

Pat is a 55-year old schoolteacher who was diagnosed with diabetes five years ago. She was substantially overweight and her blood sugar was four times normal last year, despite taking pills to lower it. Her doctor said she was going to have to start insulin if her blood sugar didn't come down. That shocked her into getting her diabetes under control. She started riding her exercise bike and worked at staying on a 1200-calorie diet.

What made following the diet especially hard was that her husband likes pastries and sweets and having those fattening, sugary foods in the house was a constant temptation.

Pat's husband didn't understand why she was making such a big deal about needing to lose weight. He thought she looked fine and she didn't seem sick.

Finally, in late January, Pat got tired of her husband's lack of support for her diabetes program. She found a community evening class on diabetes and brought him along. A good portion of the class dealt with nutrition, especially the importance of avoiding food high in fat and sugar. He said the class was interesting.

The next morning he offered her jelly donuts—and was surprised at her refusal!

Despite the slow start, Pat's husband eventually did help. The first change was to tell her he didn't need to have pastries and cookies in the house if that made it harder for her to stay on her diet. The second change was to agree to walk with Pat almost every day.

The changes have brought results. Pat lost thirty pounds in eight months and she credits a good deal of that success to her husband's support and cooperation.

John's Story

John is a 39-year old draftsman who also has diabetes. He was only 9 when he got it and he's had it for 30 years. He injects insulin three times a day, eats meals at scheduled times, avoids sugary foods, exercises every day, and carries candy or other snacks in case his blood sugar gets too low. He also tests his blood sugar five to seven times a day and carries the equipment he needs to do that, plus extra insulin.

John is divorced and lives alone. He often feels that his co-workers and the people he knows socially don't care about his diabetes. At office parties his colleagues only bring foods he can't eat and nobody pays attention when he tells them that he needs to eat at a certain time.

He doesn't have any of the serious complications that some people with diabetes get after 30 years, but he worries about what still might happen. He hasn't escaped completely unscathed, though. He feels tired and sick when his blood sugar is out of control and often feels sick and tired of being different and having to pay attention to his diabetes. Diabetes is expensive too–John spends $150-$250 a month just for his supplies.

Pat and John Have Different Kinds of Diabetes

Pat and John got diabetes at different ages. Pat was middle-aged. John was a child. They also have some very different ways they take care of their diabetes. Pat takes pills, while John takes insulin. Pat still needs to lose some weight, John doesn't.

Type 2 Diabetes

Pat has type 2 diabetes, which used to be called adult onset diabetes or non-insulin-dependent diabetes. She doesn't need insulin because she is still making some of her own. About 90-95% of the people with diabetes have the kind Pat has. They got it as older adults.

Type 1 Diabetes

John has type 1 diabetes, which used to be called juvenile onset diabetes, insulin-dependent diabetes, or brittle diabetes. Five to ten percent of the people with diabetes have type 1.

What They Have In Common

What Pat and John *do* have in common is that they both need to take steps to keep their blood sugar at normal levels. Also, they could both get the same serious diabetes complications. Lastly, they share a chronic disease that, unless some wonderful cure comes along, will require management for the rest of their lives.

Common Misunderstandings

To help the Pat or John in your life, you may need to unlearn some things about diabetes. Most people think that there are only two things a person with diabetes has to do:

1. Avoid food with sugar.
2. Take insulin shots.

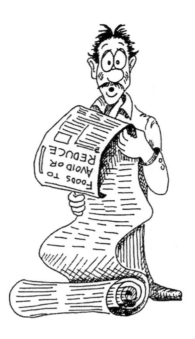

But John eats candy or some form of sugar when his blood sugar gets too low and most people with diabetes don't take insulin shots.

There is a lot more to diabetes than sugar and shots. If you already know more than this, you are better informed about diabetes than 90% of the American public. That's according to the people with diabetes who tell me what their friends and family members know–or think they know.

Most Diabetes "Teachers" Have Diabetes

The burden of educating people who don't have diabetes has been left almost entirely to the people who have it. Only at social or athletic events do non-diabetics see people with diabetes test or ask for a special food or drink. Then their interest and curiosity are piqued, leading to questions or comments. Some people with diabetes tell me they don't mind telling other people about their disease, while others just want to be left alone to do their diabetes tasks without inquiring minds or offers of help.

Some diabetics[1] tell a friend or family member what they need to know to help keep them safe but that's all they share. They are the exceptions, though. Almost all of the people with diabetes I've spoken or written to, say it would be a help if others knew more. That's why over 300 people (from 11 countries) with diabetes answered my questions about what they wished other people knew about living with diabetes. They told me about the things they hate. High on their lists were: worrying about complications, pricking a finger for a blood test, taking insulin, and paying for supplies. Happily, they had an even longer list of ways their family members, friends, and colleagues make it easier for them to handle their diabetes.

They don't all agree on how they want you to treat them. Some of them want you to treat them like anyone else. Others are pleased and appreciative when you provide special food or ask them how they are doing. It's not hard to learn which of these approaches you should adopt with your loved one, friend or co-worker. Just ask.

This Book Will Get You Started

This book is a guide to those of us who don't have diabetes from those who live with it every waking and sleeping hour.

In addition to the people with diabetes who shared their stories for this book, I have 20+ years experience as a registered nurse and diabetes educator helping people with diabetes. My interest started during nursing school when one of my first patients was 45-year old Beverly who was in the hospital to have her foot amputated. Her caring husband was there every day, patting her hand and bringing her what comfort he could. I was so sad for both of them. And, young know-it-all that I was, I thought, "If only someone had told Beverly not to eat sugar and to take her insulin every day, she wouldn't be suffering this tragedy." Little did I then know how much more complicated diabetes care is and that even if she had

---

[1] Some people consider it politically incorrect to call a person with diabetes a "diabetic." They prefer "a person with diabetes" to avoid giving the idea that the person is just a disease and not a whole person. However, almost everyone uses "diabetic" in conversation, even those with diabetes. Only two people of the hundreds I asked resented being called a diabetic. In this book, I use both terms.

followed those beliefs faithfully, she would, quite possibly, still have needed the amputation.

Fast forward to more years of taking care of people in the hospital and in their homes while I was a visiting nurse. Many of my patients experienced life-changing diabetes complications. I very much wanted to *prevent* some of that distress. So I became a Certified Diabetes Educator.

It was clear from my first meeting with Beverly and all the patients I've had since, that family members and friends have a tremendous impact on how people with diabetes deal with their disease. So this book was born.

Although someone with diabetes may find parts of this book interesting and the news about recent developments as well as recipes useful, it's not meant to be a comprehensive guide to diabetes management for the person with diabetes or for a person taking total care of a dependent person with diabetes. Your best resource for detailed management is your, or your loved one's, physician and diabetes care team. Still, the Suggested Reading List in the Appendix, has some diabetes books and magazines you may find additionally helpful.

Since there are different types of diabetes and because your relationship with the person with diabetes may be casual, friendly, or intimate, and because people with diabetes are just as different as you and I, there is often no single right way to handle each situation.

That's why there is some background about diabetes with general medical information in most chapters, followed by suggestions picked up from years of listening to people with diabetes talk about what they wished their friends and family members knew. Included are specific ways in which you can help the person with diabetes, whether by action or by providing emotional support.

Because some readers may want to read the chapters out of order, some basic explanatory material is briefly repeated.

Also, since many of you may be relatives of people with diabetes and may worry that you could get it, there is a chapter called *Do I Have It? Will I Get It?* Actually you could get it even if you aren't related to someone with diabetes.

I've included some of my favorite low-sugar and low-fat recipes, and I also urge you to buy a diabetes cookbook or two or check out recent ones at the library with more selections; the ones in this book are just a start to get you through a few meals and to be able to bring healthy treats to a social gathering.

The Appendix has a thorough glossary (so you won't need to write down definitions as you go along).

People with diabetes can learn to live well with their disease. John has, despite not having anyone to help with his diabetes anymore. He's learned to do it all himself. And that's hard. He'd love to have someone give some thought to his need to eat on time and avoid sweets. He'd probably love to have you for a friend or office mate after you've read this book.

That's because with your understanding, cooperation, and support you can make an important and positive difference in the care people with diabetes take of themselves. Pat's husband has made that difference.

2

A Short History of Diabetes

The Years Before Insulin

A scribe in Egypt 3,500 years ago described the disease that we know today as diabetes.

The Greeks later called the condition *diabetes mellitus* meaning "honey siphon:" "siphon" because of the sufferer's unending urination and "honey" because the urine was sweet tasting. (You don't want to know how they knew it was sweet but doctors nowadays must be grateful to have labs to send urine specimens to.)

In those days, young people who got diabetes wasted away to skin and bones despite ravenous appetites and voracious eating. They urinated a lot because they drank huge amounts of water, but they were still thirsty and wanted more. They got infections that wouldn't clear up, and they became progressively weaker. The only treatment that kept young people alive for a year or two, and older patients alive for longer periods, was a starvation diet. The recommended diet had 500 calories, almost all of that fat and protein, with almost no starches or sugars. Physicians didn't know why that worked, but the less starch and sugar their patients ate, the less sugar they lost in their urine and the slower their weight plunged.

For centuries doctors thought diabetes was a kidney disease. They were wrong about that and really had no clue as to the cause of diabetes until 1890, when Joseph von Mering and Oskar Minkowsky showed that in animals, removal of the pancreas caused diabetes. They believed that the pancreas produced a substance that controlled the metabolism of food, especially sugars and starches (carbohydrates).

Two decades earlier, Paul Langerhans had described groups of cells in the pancreas, subsequently named the islets of Langerhans, but no one appreciated their importance at the time.

A Baltimore pathologist, E. L. Opie, noticed that in the pancreas of a young woman who had died of diabetes, the islets described by Langerhans were shriveled up.

Given what was known, it seemed logical that if you ground up a pancreas, made a solution, and gave it to experimental animals with diabetes, they might be cured. They tried that but the animals still died of diabetes.

The problem was that the pancreas doesn't produce just the special something that prevents diabetes. It also manufactures digestive enzymes (powerful chemicals that *go through a duct into the intestines* to help digest food). In the pancreas, the clumps of cells that produce enzymes and the ones that produce the "diabetes substance" are separate.

What those early diabetes researchers didn't know is that the "magical" substance *they were looking for goes directly into the blood.* In our bodies, it never comes in contact with the digestive enzymes the pancreas also makes, so it has no need for protection against those caustic chemicals. By grinding up the whole pancreas, early researchers exposed the vulnerable substance they were looking for to digestive enzymes which destroyed it.

The Discovery of Insulin

In 1921 a young Canadian orthopedic surgeon and medical school instructor with time on his hands, read all the available information about diabetes. He was trying to make sense for his medical students of the many conflicting ideas about diabetes. He also had a personal interest–his childhood sweetheart had died of diabetes when the young physician was fifteen years old.

That tragedy was why the 29-year old Canadian, who had begun his university studies in theology to please his parents, switched to medicine in his sophomore year. He graduated as a physician in 1916 and was immediately sent to a field hospital in France. He became a fine surgeon there, was wounded, and showed great compassion for his patients by continuing to operate despite his own injury. He came close to bleeding to death and later almost lost an arm to gangrene. After the war, he returned to Canada to start his private practice. To earn enough to survive, he taught physiology to medical students at the University of Western Ontario.

His name was Frederick Banting and he would get the Nobel Prize for the discovery that changed the treatment of diabetes and brought hope to thousands of its sufferers–the discovery of insulin.

While preparing a class on the pancreas, Banting reviewed von Mering's and Minkowski's work and that of all the other scientists who had contributed what little was known about diabetes. He developed some ideas about how the elusive substance in the pancreas might be found, separated, and used in treatment.

His own colleagues at the University of Western Ontario were not interested in expending resources for such a risky project, but they encouraged Banting to see Dr. J.J.R. Macleod, a renowned expert in diabetes, at the University of Toronto.

Banting made the long, cold trip to Toronto to beg Dr. Macleod to help with his idea for separating the substances of the pancreas, but Macleod turned him down. Macleod thought it ridiculous that a young doctor with no research experience should tread where great men had failed. Banting persevered, however, and finally Macleod, who was going away on vacation in the summer of 1921, reluctantly allowed Banting the use of a lab, ten laboratory dogs, and the unpaid help of a research assistant for the two months he would be away.

Charles Best, the research assistant, had just graduated with a bachelor's degree in biochemistry. He was as interested as Banting in finding a cure for diabetes because he had lost a beloved aunt to the disease. Banting and Best pooled their savings of less than $500 and on May 17, 1921, they went to work.

They scrimped on food, used up their money for more dogs and supplies, suffered in the hot lab, and made history. These special men–Banting, skilled in surgical techniques, and Best, educated in chemical processes–despite every difficulty imaginable, produced what they were looking for in only two months.

Banting tied off the tiny pancreas ducts through which digestive enzymes go to the intestines. The enzymes backed up, causing the enzyme cells to shrivel and die. Six weeks later, when Banting removed the pancreas, only insulin-producing islets were functioning.

On July 27, 1921, Banting and Best injected the substance they had isolated from the islets into a comatose dog that was dying of diabetes. In hours, the dog was up, energetic, and with no sugar in its urine, but the next day it again lapsed into a diabetic coma and died. Banting and Best then knew that they needed a continuous supply of this miraculous substance, but they also knew that they weren't going to get enough of it from a few dogs. They would need the limitless supply of pancreases they could get from livestock.

To get money to keep their experiments going, Banting sold his car. This meant his and Best's dozens of trips to stockyards to buy ox pancreases had to be made by streetcar. Keeping the pancreases cool and unspoiled on the slow, hot trips was difficult but Banting and Best got the organs back to the lab safely and were able to extract the precious insulin.

After trying insulin on each other with no ill effects, Banting and Best felt ready to start helping the dozens of dying victims of diabetes in Toronto's hospitals. "Not so fast," said Professor Macleod, just back from his vacation. He was not amused that the two young nobodies should have succeeded where renowned scientists had tried and failed for decades. He was not pleased that they hadn't learned a lesson in humility. Macleod, a recognized expert in diabetes, made them prove everything all over again to his satisfaction.

Happily, everything went well, and Macleod, instead of further blocking Banting and Best's work, took up the banner to get insulin improved and recognized. He appointed a chemist, James Collip, to help further purify the substance, he changed the name from *isletin* (named after the islets of Langerhans) to the more easily pronounced insulin, and finally, in January 1922, he approved the first testing of insulin on a human.

A mere six months after the lab dog had been briefly revived, a young boy dying of diabetes in a Toronto hospital was offered the chance to be the first person to be treated with insulin. He was bedridden and near death when he and his parents accepted Banting's offer. Within a day, the boy was miraculously better. He was given an injection of insulin every day and was quickly joined by other patients Banting treated.

Meanwhile, Professor Macleod traveled around Canada and the United States telling physicians and scientists about his team's miraculous discovery of insulin. He gave Banting and Best little credit, though he acknowledged Collip's work in purifying insulin.

In 1923, Banting and Macleod were awarded the Nobel Prize for medical research. Banting was furious that Macleod was acknowledged and Best was not. He threatened to refuse the prize but eventually accepted, and gave half of his prize money to Best.

Insulin did not cure diabetes, but it lengthened lives and improved the quality of those lives. The young boy who was first treated with insulin died 13 years later of pneumonia and complications of diabetes. He would have died in a matter of days or, at most, a couple of weeks if Banting had not had insulin to give him.

The University of Toronto received a patent for insulin. Although the university never charged drug companies for the use of the process to extract insulin, it did charge a fee to test the purity and activity of the insulin the companies marketed. Profit from the fees went to fund further research by Banting, Best, and Collip.

By the end of 1923, just a little over two years after Banting and Best's first success with the dog, insulin was available in medical centers all over the world. What had once been a rapidly fatal disease to children and young adults had an effective treatment.

Insulin still doesn't cure diabetes. It, and the oral medicines since developed for type 2 diabetes, only help control the disease. Diabetes needs careful managing for its sufferers to reap the maximum benefit from Frederick Banting and Charles Best's marvelous work.

Other Treatment Discoveries

Wonderful as insulin was, it couldn't do everything. Doctors and patients still needed to find the right combination of insulin and food. To do that, they needed to know their blood sugar level as accurately as possible. Remember the physicians in ancient times that used to taste urine as a test for sugar?

Testing for Sugar

Urine Tests

Tasting was eventually followed by the Benedict test–considered the state of the art in its time. It required placing some urine in a test-tube, adding Benedict solution (a blue fluid), and warming the test-tube in a pan of boiling water. After five minutes, the color of the mixture showed whether sugar was in the urine. More than soup got cooked in the kitchens of people with diabetes.

Urine testing continued to get easier. First the cooking became unnecessary–it was replaced by merely dropping a tablet into a urine sample. Finally, the urine test strip for sugar became available. All this test needed was to hold a chemically treated strip in a stream of urine, shake off the excess, and match the color on the strip to the color chart on the package of strips. This test was easy but it still wasn't very accurate.

For decades, people with diabetes and their physicians based diabetes treatment on home urine sugar tests and occasional laboratory urine and blood tests. But urine tests for sugar give information that can be hours old (while the urine is stored in the bladder) and only indicate high levels, since urine tests can't detect lows.

Blood Tests

Home blood glucose (sugar) testing was a wonderful advance in diabetes treatment. Blood tests identified low, normal, and high blood sugar and gave an immediate result, not one that was hours old. To perform this test, the person pricked a finger, placed a drop of blood on a chemically treated strip, waited one minute, wiped off the strip, waited another minute, and then held the strip up to a color chart on the package just as was done with the urine test strips. With the blood test strip, the person testing knew within 60mg/dl (a significant range since normal blood sugar is about 80-120 mg/dl) what his or her blood sugar was two minutes earlier.

The next improvement and current technology was the blood sugar meter, which can give a specific level of blood sugar like 127, instead of a range of from 120-180.

Improvements in Insulin

Insulin, too, changed from what Banting and Best collected from animal pancreases. Beef and pork insulins frequently caused allergic reactions at the injection site that could lessen their effectiveness. They are no longer made or sold in the U.S. Almost all insulin used in the world today is synthetic human insulin made in laboratories.

Back in 1922, there was only one strength of insulin, similar to the regular insulin used today. Its action wore off quickly so several daily injections were necessary. Fifteen years after regular insulin became available, a Danish research team headed by H. C. Hagedorn found a combination of insulin with a substance called protamine that slowed insulin's absorption from the tissues. Eventually, mixtures with zinc were developed that were so slowly absorbed that many people got by with only one injection a day.

But the newest research shows that one injection a day, even of long-acting insulin, does not come close to keeping blood sugar in the normal range, as a well-functioning pancreas does. People who don't make their own insulin but want the nearly normal blood sugar that helps prevent complications, are returning to taking three and four injections a day. Newer, faster-acting insulins and better slow-acting insulins have made it easier to get less variable blood sugar levels.

Though Frederick Banting and Charles Best's work has been improved upon, they are truly the heroes in the history of diabetes treatment.

3

What Does Diabetes Do?

John's Story–October, 1963

John had been feeling thirsty all the time. He drank tons of juice, soda, and water, but the thirst didn't go away. His mother noticed he was eating a lot more too. "I can't believe how much food a nine-year old boy can put away," she remarked to his father. "He sure doesn't get fat; in fact, he looks to me as if he's lost some weight."

John's father said, "He's a growing boy. What do you expect?"

John's father was wrong. It wasn't because he was a growing boy that John was eating and drinking a lot and losing weight.

In the weeks that followed, John drank more fluids than ever and went to the bathroom a lot. He also felt tired all the time, no matter how much sleep he got or how much he ate. He lost 13 pounds in four weeks.

When his mother realized how much weight he'd lost, she made an appointment with his pediatrician. After hearing the symptoms, John's doctor asked him to go to the bathroom and fill a cup with urine.

A nurse dipped a specially treated paper strip into the sample, and, sure enough, it tested very positive for sugar. The doctor wasted no time. He told John's mother that he was almost sure John had diabetes and that he needed to go to the hospital to get started on insulin.

John spent two weeks in the hospital, getting his dosage of insulin calculated. He also learned about what an insulin reaction felt like, what to eat, what not to eat, and all kinds of other information about diabetes. He even learned how to do the urine test the nurse had done in the doctor's office. Nowadays, he would have been taught how to test his blood, but that wasn't available to patients in 1963.

His mother stayed with him and anxiously tried to take it all in too. Today, nobody spends two weeks in the hospital if all they need is to adjust their insulin dosage and learn about diabetes.

One reason that long hospital stay was necessary was that in 1963 there was no way people with diabetes could test their own blood at home and have a good idea what their blood sugar was at that moment. Patients couldn't give accurate, current information to the doctor over the phone and have the doctor easily calculate a safe, effective insulin dosage. When John was newly diagnosed, doctors waited for lab results of a blood test before deciding how to adjust the amounts of insulin and food. Physicians knew that once the patient went home, they would lose the information from blood tests and have to rely on urine tests until the next office visit when blood could be sent to a lab. Of course, life in the hospital and life outside the hospital would not be the same, but that was the best that could be done back then.

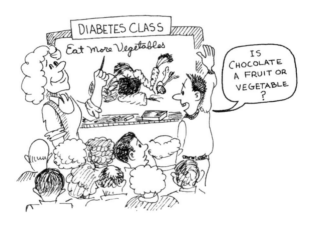

John hated the shots and hated the urine testing. He thought it was very unfair that he couldn't eat candy anymore like other kids. His mom wasn't happy either. She was given lots of pamphlets and advice about shopping, measuring food, menu planning, how to help John if his blood sugar got low, how to boil the glass syringes, and on and on.

His father wasn't as involved. He did wonder, though, why it had happened to John. No one in *his* family had diabetes and his wife said nobody on her side had it either. Wasn't diabetes a hereditary disease?

John and his family learned a lot about diabetes and how to control it, but why John got it is something no one was able to tell them. Even today, scientists have theories but no sure answers about what causes diabetes.

Here are some questions John and his folks asked and people today are still concerned about. The answers are what you'd get today from doctor and nurses:

What is diabetes?

Diabetes is a malfunction of the body's use of food that results in a person's being unable to automatically regulate the level of sugar in the blood. Diabetes affects the metabolism of carbohydrates (sugars and starches), protein, and fat but because the primary problem in diabetes is the level of blood sugar and 90% of carbohydrates are converted to sugar, carbohydrates are the main concern. To understand what goes wrong, you need to know how the body uses food, especially carbohydrates.

How is food normally used by the body?

The kind of food your body's cells prefer is sugar. Actually, it's a particular kind of sugar called glucose. Cells need glucose the way your car needs gasoline.

Most of the carbohydrate foods you swallow is changed into glucose in the small intestine and then absorbed into the blood where it's carried to every cell in the body.

But getting glucose this far is only equivalent to filling your car's gas tank. That gas still needs to get into the motor, or in the case of glucose, into every cell.

How does the glucose or sugar get into the cell?

What gets the glucose into the cell is insulin, a hormone produced by the pancreas. Hormones are substances that certain body organs produce and release into the blood and that have a specific effect in cells in other parts of the body. The pancreas not only produces the insulin and releases it into the blood, it senses when and how much is needed.

The insulin "escorts" the glucose from the blood into the cell, where it can be used as the cell's food or be stored for future use.

What happens if there is no insulin?

When there is no insulin available, the glucose stays in the blood, and cells don't get their food. When cells don't get their glucose supply, the person starts experiencing the symptoms of diabetes.

What are the symptoms of John's kind of diabetes (type 1)?

Increased hunger	Increased thirst	Abdominal pain
Weight loss	Increased urination	Leg cramps
Tiredness	Blurred vision	Headaches
Infections	Nausea and vomiting	Irritability

How can a person have increased hunger, eat more, and still lose weight?

When cells do not get the food they need, the body "thinks" it's starving. It tries to get more food by stimulating the sense of hunger. Unfortunately, eating more doesn't help because more food is just changed into glucose, which makes the blood even more sugary. When that doesn't work, the body tries to get glucose from its protein supplies, most of which are in muscle tissue. The liver then converts that protein into glucose. But, again, the glucose level in the blood just goes higher. As muscles waste away, it's possible to actually lose weight despite eating extra food.

Where does tiredness come in?

Along with the hunger and weight loss comes tiredness. Eight hours sleep, vitamin pills, pots of coffee: nothing seems to help. Cells without food are cells that don't want to move muscles.

Why do people with diabetes get more infections?

Muscle cells are not the only cells that are going without glucose, the cells in the immune system, especially white blood cells are unable to work, so germs and viruses may cause frequent, slow-healing infections.

Not only are the infection-fighting cells starving from lack of glucose, excess glucose in the blood is an ideal feeding and breeding ground for many bacteria and fungi. That's why vaginal and urinary tract infections are common at the time diabetes is diagnosed or any other time when blood sugar stays high for too long.

Why does diabetes make a person feel thirsty and urinate more?

Without insulin, the blood glucose level can rise to 10 times normal. Since even a little more than the normal range is harmful, the body tries to get rid of the excess glucose. The kidneys try to flush it out by making more urine. Thirst is increased to get more water for the kidneys' increased urine production. The person drinks more and urinates more. This urine has a lot of glucose in it. In fact, this is where much of the glucose that couldn't get into the cells goes.

Losing fluid and calories in the urine is another cause of weight loss.

The body's attempt to get rid of the sugar by making sweet urine is still not enough to get the blood sugar to normal levels. The kidneys only start making extra urine when the glucose in the blood is about double the normal level, which is too high to maintain a healthy cell environment. To lower it further requires a change in diet, exercise, and, often, medication.

Why is blurred vision a symptom of diabetes?
What does sugar in the blood have to do with eyesight?

High sugar levels in the blood change the shape and flexibility of lens so it's unable to focus an image precisely on the retina at the back of the eye. This causes blurred vision. The good news is that this blurring is not permanent. Within several weeks of getting blood sugar under control, vision is as sharp as it was before. The bad news is that permanent damage can be done to the retina at the back of the eye if blood sugar levels are high for years.

Who gets type 1 diabetes?

Type 1 diabetes is most often first diagnosed in children and young adults.

What other types of diabetes are there?

Type 2 diabetes is the most common type of diabetes. It occurs when the pancreas produces some insulin, but perhaps not quite enough, or when the insulin is not being used effectively. It progresses more slowly and may not have the dramatic symptoms of type 1 diabetes. It is more common in people over 40, although children or young adults can also get it.

Some pregnant women get a diabetes called gestational diabetes. It's due to the effect of pregnancy hormones that disturb the usual balance of food and insulin. It's temporary in more than 90% of women who get it, though it usually recurs in any subsequent pregnancies and, not infrequently, can return later in life as type 2 diabetes.

Latent Autoimmune Diabetes in Adults (LADA) or type 1.5 diabetes is a form of type 1 diabetes, but because people are older than 25 or 30 when they are diagnosed, it's often assumed to be type 2. In fact, initially, they usually do well with a diabetes meal plan and may not even need diabetes pills. Within months, however, they usually need insulin.

There are also other kinds of diabetes due to disease of the pancreas or its surgical removal, glandular problems, and medications that raise blood sugar, such as cortisone. These conditions either decrease or eliminate the supply of insulin or make it less effective.

Does eating sugar cause diabetes?

No. If a person does not have diabetes, the pancreas can produce enough insulin, so that any amount of sugar will be used effectively or stored as fat.

Is diabetes contagious?

No. It is not at all like a cold or the measles.

What causes diabetes?

Diabetes is caused by both heredity and environment. Type 1, the kind John has, is believed to be caused by a genetic defect that predisposes an individual's immune system to overreact to a virus.

Perhaps some other stress to the immune system is also involved. When these factors are present, the insulin-producing cells of the pancreas may be destroyed.

Type 2 diabetes is more likely to occur in a person who has other family members with type 2. Frequently the pancreas is pumping out lots of insulin but the cells "resist" the insulin. Excess body fat is usually at least partly to blame for that resistance. In fact, eight out of ten people with type 2 diabetes are overweight.

Along with heredity and excess body fat, there is a another contributing cause to diabetes: stress. Actually, both viruses and excess fat are stresses to the body, but we usually think of stress as a psychological burden. When we lose a loved one, a job, or our health, we call that stress. If too much is expected of us, we experience stress. But *any* change in our lives including illness is a stress that requires the body to adapt.

The body tries to cope with stress with three hormones: adrenaline (epinephrine), cortisol (similar to cortisone), and insulin. All three make it easier for us to flee or fight some danger in our surroundings. Adrenaline raises the blood pressure and heart rate so our muscles can get extra blood to run or fight. Cortisol helps the body change stored protein and fat into sugar for use by the muscles as fuel. And insulin gets that sugar into the muscle cells.

If everything works well, escaping or fighting uses up the sugar, and when the danger is over, the body returns to is normal state. Temporary stress is normal in life, and our bodies are well equipped to handle it. But too much for too long can overtax the body's coping mechanisms. If stress continues at high levels, the extra blood sugar that the cortisol calls up may be more than some strained pancreases can handle. If not enough insulin can be made or if insulin resistance is present, high blood sugar becomes constant and diabetes results.

What happens if someone with type 1 doesn't take insulin?

Because insulin is so essential to the body's survival, a complete lack of it, or even a seriously low level causing continuously rising blood sugar, rapidly causes tiredness, hunger, weight loss, infections, increased thirst, increased urination, and blurred vision. In days, or at most a couple of weeks, people with type 1 diabetes start reporting all or almost all of these symptoms. If they do not get diagnosed and get insulin, they eventually lapse into a coma and die.

Some people with diabetes take pills instead of insulin, why can't John?

Blood sugar lowering pills require that the pancreas produce a significant amount of insulin. John is producing no insulin. This is evident because when his urine was tested, it contained two things that shouldn't have been there: sugar and ketones. Anybody with diabetes can have sugar in their urine, but ketones, a waste product of burning fat, are almost always a sign that the person has a severe shortage of insulin–so severe that the body is unable to use the sugar in the blood and must burn stored fat to try to survive.

How is the onset of type 2 diabetes different?

A person with undiagnosed type 2 diabetes will often complain of tiredness. But since tiredness is such a common feeling, it can be overlooked as a symptom of diabetes, even by a doctor . People just think, "Of course I'm tired. I'm getting old."

Type 2 comes on so slowly that some people have type 2 for five or more years before it's diagnosed. They may actually suffer a complication–such as an infection that doesn't heal, leg pain, or numb feet. The doctor visit to treat the complication may be when they find out they have diabetes.

What are some common symptoms of type 2 diabetes?

> Tiredness or drowsiness
> Blurred vision
> Tingling, numbness, or pain in legs or feet
> Slow healing cuts and sores
> Frequent skin infections or itchy skin

What are the complications of diabetes?

The complications most people think about first are blindness, kidney failure, and foot amputations. These are the end results of damage to the retina of the eye, the kidney, and the nerves and blood vessels in the legs.

People are less likely to associate heart attacks and strokes with diabetes, but years of high blood sugar together with high cholesterol levels in the blood can lead to a build-up of plaque inside blood vessels.

In one hospital I worked in, there were more patients with diabetes in the cardiac unit than in the diabetes unit.

Nerves in many parts of the body can be damaged and are the basis for complications ranging from mild to life threatening.

How Can Complications Be Avoided?

The most important factor in avoiding diabetic complications is to keep blood sugar levels close to normal.

American Diabetes Association Recommended goals:

	Fasting	2 hours after meals*	A1c**
ADA	70-130 mg/dl	under 180	under 7%

* Start timing with 1st bite of food
** The A1c is a lab test that shows approximately the average blood sugar the last 3 months. Normal is 4-6%.

What are the main differences between type 1 and type 2?

Here is an overview of the similarities and differences in the two main types of diabetes:

	Type 2	Type 1
Number of US cases (2008)	About 22 million	About 2 million
Age when *usually* diagnosed	Over 40	Under 40
Speed of onset	Weeks to years	Days to weeks
Need to take insulin	Sometimes	Always
Can treat with pills	Often	Never
Diet and exercise part of treatment	Always	Always
Can get complications	Yes	Yes

Is there a cure for diabetes?

At present there are three treatments for diabetes that prove to be cures for some of the people who undergo them. The first two are transplant procedures for those with type 1 diabetes.

1. The oldest "cure" is a whole or partial pancreas transplant. Such transplants are done in only a few medical centers. Pancreas transplants require expensive lifelong immunosuppressive drugs to prevent rejection of the new organ. The surgery and the medications required afterward are, at best, only partially reimbursed by insurance. Frequently, companies refuse to pay any part of the expense on the grounds that pancreas transplants are experimental.

2. More recently, some centers are trying to transplant only the cells that make insulin instead of the whole pancreas. These islet cell transplants are not surgery but an injection of cells from a cadaver pancreas into the portal vein of the liver where it's hoped they will grow and produce insulin in response to sugar in the blood. The procedure takes about 15 minutes. These transplants are also considered experimental.

For most people with diabetes, neither of these options is possible because of the anti-rejection drug side effects (including kidney damage), the huge expense, and the limited pool of cadaver pancreases. And few patients remain insulin-free after a few years.

3. The third option is abdominal surgery for weight loss. This is for obese patients with type 2 diabetes. Some procedures make the stomach smaller, others bypass part of the gastrointestinal system. The goal is mainly to modify the ability of the stomach and/or intestines to absorb nutrients.

These procedures don't require anti-rejection drugs since no tissue is transplanted.

Intestinal surgery dramatically improves blood sugar levels but is not without risks so most centers only accept extremely obese patients who are at considerable risk of cardiovascular and other complications. After surgery, a rigorous diet of small meals plus vitamin supplements is essential. Since these are relatively new procedures, it's not yet known if the improvements last beyond a few years. More long term studies are needed.

The work being done with these treatments plus research on stem cells suggest that progress is being made and we that can reasonably hope for a cure in the future.

Does diabetes ever go away by itself?

No, but there may be a temporary remission.

In people with type 2 diabetes who are overweight and sedentary, lifestyle changes such as healthy eating and vigorous exercise six or seven days a week can result in a return to normal blood sugar levels in the first years after they're diagnosed. Happily, maintaining normal blood sugar reduces their risk for future diabetes complications to about the same as a non-diabetic. Unfortunately, it doesn't take away the original inherited defect so a return to old habits or the stress of an illness can result in high blood sugar again.

In about 20% of recently diagnosed people with type 1 diabetes, the need for injected insulin may decrease or even stop for a short while. Usually this "honeymoon phase" lasts a few weeks, although there have been a few cases in which it continued for two or more years before the insulin dosage had to be increased or restarted.

One theory about why this occurs is that in some people at the time of diagnosis, the insulin-producing cells that are not yet dead, are too exhausted to carry the full load formerly borne by millions of healthy cells. These "exhausted" cells no longer produce insulin. However, after a few weeks of insulin injections during which no demands are being placed on the pancreas' beta cells, they get a "second wind" and can produce enough, or nearly enough, insulin without injections–for a while.

Cases of people in the "honeymoon phase" are probably responsible for reports of miraculous "cures" and successes with alternate therapies. The news of someone going off insulin is a much bigger story than the person's eventual relapse, so you probably would never hear that insulin later was needed again–permanently.

4

Treatments:
Different Pokes for Different Folks

John has type 1 diabetes and takes insulin three times a day. But even though everyone with type 1 needs insulin, not everyone takes three injections a day.

Pat, whom you also met in Chapter 1, has type 2 diabetes. There is even more variation in the treatment of her kind of diabetes. Some people with type 2, like Pat, take pills to help reduce their blood sugar. Others need insulin, and still others control their disease with diet and exercise alone.

What makes the difference? What else do people do to control their disease?

Here are questions that Pat, John, or John's parents asked at one time or another about treating diabetes.

How often do people with type 1 need insulin?

People with very little or no insulin production need to inject insulin several times a day or use an insulin pump (see Chapter 5). At present, there is no other way to get insulin reliably into the body. When insulin was a new medicine, there was only one kind, which we now call regular insulin. Its effects lasted only a few hours, so several injections were necessary every day. Later, insulin was also formulated into long-lasting and intermediate-acting types that can lower the blood glucose for many hours, so the treatment swung in the other direction to one injection a day. Even though one shot per day might be enough to prevent the symptoms of very high blood sugar, it really didn't reproduce the varying insulin levels a normal pancreas produces throughout the day. Type 1s had rigid meal and snack times and frequently got too low. People didn't appreciate how inadequate this one shot was because urine testing didn't show the true blood sugar levels.

Today, most people with type 1 take four injections a day, a rapid-acting insulin before meals and a long-lasting insulin at bedtime that works about 24 hours. This comes closer to what a normal pancreas does: it gives a surge of insulin with meals and a drop every few minutes the rest of the time.

How is the treatment for type 2 diabetes different?

People with type 2 diabetes produce their own insulin. It may not be quite enough or it may not be used efficiently, but they are not experiencing a complete absence of insulin. Still, they may have one or more of several other problems.

1. One problem has to do with an incorrect signal being given to the liver. In people without diabetes, when insulin and blood sugar levels are high (*after meals*, for example), the liver removes some glucose from the blood, and stores it in a form called glycogen. When the insulin level is low and blood sugar is lower, as it typically is *between meals*, another hormone produced by the pancreas, called glucagon, signals the liver to break down the stored glycogen, turn it back into glucose, and release it into the bloodstream to prevent blood sugar from going too low.

In type 2 diabetes, the pancreas may continue to release glucagon even *shortly after a meal*, causing the liver to release glucose when levels are already high. Adding that glucose to the glucose from the food means that the blood sugar goes up even higher. A properly functioning pancreas would regulate this process, but in type 2, it may fail to do so. Metformin (Glucophage) is a commonly pre-scribed pill that acts on the liver to reduce the release of glucose.

2. If the pancreas can no longer produce enough insulin naturally to get glucose into cells the solution may be pills called sulfonyl-ureas. They cause the pancreas to produce more insulin. Common ones are glipizide (Glucotrol), glyburide (Glynase, Micronase, and DiaBeta) and glimepiride (Amaryl).

3. The third possible problem of type 2 diabetes may be that insulin is not released quickly enough after eating. Usually, getting

the new batch of glucose from the meal out of the blood and into the cells should take no more than three hours. If the insulin release is delayed, the blood sugar stays high longer than it should. Alpha-glucosidase inhibitors (acarbose [Precose] and miglitol [Glyset]) pills slow down the digestion of carbohydrates so a poky pancreas has a chance to keep up.

4. The fourth problem is resistance to insulin in the muscles and liver. A person could produce plenty of insulin and still have high blood sugar and feel lack of energy if this were the problem. Thiazolidinedione pills (pioglitazone [Actos] and rosiglitazone [Avandia]) reduce this resistance.

5. If the problem is a combination of insufficient insulin production *and* excessive liver glucose production, two new pills (DPP-4 inhibitors), sitagliptin (Januvia) and saxagliptin (Onglyza), may be considered.

6. Exenatide (Byetta) is a relatively new injected medication with several actions: it enhances insulin secretion when blood sugar is high, decreases liver's glucose output, and may suppress appetite thereby leading to weight loss. The last effect has made this a popular drug (despite being an injection) for people who want to lose weight.

Are medications always necessary for type 2 diabetes?

Changes in lifestyle can lessen insulin resistance and help the body's natural insulin work more efficiently. One of these changes is to lose excess weight. Another is to reduce the quantity of food and choose foods with less concentrated carbohydrate, for example, an apple instead of a candy bar. That means smaller, more frequent meals with little or no sweets or otherwise reducing carbohydrates (see Chapters 6 and 7). Exercise is the fourth beneficial change. If diet, weight loss, and exercise sufficiently reduce the need for more insulin at meals or reduce insulin resistance and the body's insulin keeps blood sugar in the normal range, no pills or shots are needed.

Why do some people with type 2 take insulin?

If, for whatever reason, the blood sugar overtime starts creeping up while taking two or three pills at their maximum dosage, insulin is the next step. For people with type 2 diabetes, one injection a day (or possibly two) may be enough to help the pancreas so that it can manage to keep blood sugar under control the rest of the time.

Many people resist taking insulin for several reasons. Some believe insulin causes complications. They've seen a loved one start taking insulin and shortly after have a foot amputated. The insulin wasn't to blame. The problem was that their relative didn't start taking insulin months or years *earlier* in time to stop the damage of high sugar levels.

Second, they may think an insulin shot is painful. It's actually almost pain free–nothing like a flu shot or most other shots.

Another reason they resist is that they may believe it is a punishment from the doctor for their inability to follow his orders such as to lose excess weight. They may have had good results from pills for years even though it was necessary for the doctor to increase the dosage and add new pills from time to time to keep their blood sugar near normal limits. Still, most patients accept taking a few more pills as a minor inconvenience and expense.

But then the day comes when the patient is taking the maximum dosage of the medicine, his blood sugar creeps higher and higher over time, and the doctor says, "The pills aren't working. We'll have to go to insulin."

The patient's response is, "Well, they worked in the past and all you did was prescribe more pills, so do it again."

The problem is that exceeding the maximum dosage won't work. The situation is similar to taking aspirin for a headache. Just because two tablets work for the usual headache, taking 20 won't relieve the agony of a migraine. No amount of aspirin would be effective for that degree of pain, and taking 20 tablets would be toxic besides. More is not always better.

Insulin may be temporarily needed if the person is hospitalized for a heart attack, some non-diabetes related condition, or surgery. In such a case, the person with diabetes could be back on just diet and exercise in a matter of a few weeks.

Type 2, however, is a progressive disease so the tendency is to need more medicine every few years. The longer someone has diabetes, the greater the odds that they will eventually need insulin.

Will someone with type 2 become type 1 if they use insulin?

There is a common misunderstanding about the difference between type 1 and type 2 diabetes. You know by now that all people with type 1 diabetes *must* take insulin. Another description for their condition is *insulin-dependent* diabetes.

But many people with type 2 diabetes who eventually must take insulin believe that they have become transformed into type 1 diabetics. This is almost never the case. They have become insulin-*requiring* but are not insulin-*dependent*. There is a difference. They need some insulin to keep their blood sugar in the normal range, but without it they would live for months and even years. They would feel unwell, and they'd develop complications faster than if their blood sugar were within normal limits. If they got an infection, they might develop dangerously high blood sugar and become dehydrated enough to require hospitalization. But without insulin they wouldn't necessarily die in a few days or weeks. That's the difference. A person with type 1 diabetes will die in a short time without insulin.

How does the doctor know if a person needs pills or insulin and how much?

The decisions of what medicine is best, are based on the patient's blood sugar level. Blood sugar tests used to be done only occasionally. Doctors used to draw a patient's blood from a vein during an office visit and send it to a laboratory. A day or so later, the patient and doctor would know what the blood sugar was *at the time it was drawn.* Imagine having to take your car to your mechanic every time you wanted to know if it needed gas and having to wait a day or two to find out how much.

Nowadays, patients can test their own blood sugar levels several times a day instead of only a few times a year. That means that they can test at home, get the results in seconds, keep track of the results, and phone, fax, or e-mail their physician with the levels, allowing the doctor to change the dosage more frequently and to base the change on more than a single office visit and lab test. Knowing *when* blood sugar is high or low is as important as knowing the level. Diabetes management has improved enormously since patients have been able to test their own blood whenever they want to and wherever they are.

Whether the person with diabetes is three or eighty-three, has type 1 or type 2, uses insulin or takes pills, the ability to test blood sugar and make adjustments means that he or she can maintain a much more normal blood glucose. Even if the person takes neither pills nor insulin, a rising blood sugar can be an early signal that there is an infection or some other body stress occurring, or it can simply mean that pills or insulin are now needed. In either case, the physician can be called and whatever is necessary can be done–early.

Why is it important to know when blood sugar is getting low?

Since it's high blood sugar that causes long-term complications, a lower-than-normal blood sugar may sound like a good thing. But it is neither healthy nor comfortable. Low blood sugar means there isn't enough sugar in the blood so the cells aren't getting enough, which brings on unpleasant symptoms such as sweatiness, shakiness, and hunger, that signal the sugar shortage.

A low blood sugar can even be *life threatening if the brain becomes so deprived of glucose that the person becomes unconscious or has an accident. Continued brain cell deprivation can even cause a fatal coma.* Very low blood sugar is so serious that the pancreas produces a hormone called glucagon to try to correct the problem. Glucagon tells the liver to release stored glucose when the supply in the blood is low. People with diabetes don't usually rely on this emergency backup. At the first sign of sweatiness, shakiness or hunger, they eat or drink something with sugar *fast*. (See Chapter 9 on low blood sugar and how to help.)

When people had only urine tests to check for sugar, they never knew if they were getting into the low range. Lows were frequently an unpleasant surprise and, as mentioned above, could be dangerous. So it was a real boon when a test came along that accurately showed highs *and* lows and that when repeated after a few minutes, could give an idea of what direction the blood sugar was moving.

It's Hard to Compare Treatments

People with diabetes tell me they are frequently challenged by their friends and family with statements like "George has diabetes and his doctor doesn't tell him to ____." You fill in the blank. But George's doctor may have different goals for George, or George may have a problem only he and his doctor and family know about, or George may not be telling you what his doctor *really* told him to do.

Given the many treatment choices, it is not useful to compare and challenge the doctor's instructions to your friend or family member who has diabetes with anyone else's diabetes management. Here are four doctors and their patients, each with a different treatment plan.

Four Doctors: Four Treatment Plans

Doctor Smith puts most of her newly diagnosed type 2 patients on a weight loss diet before she starts them on any diabetes medication. She has them check their blood sugar daily before breakfast.

Dr. Jones prescribes oral medication for patients newly diagnosed with type 2 diabetes and sends them to a dietitian for instruction on a diet with limited portions and no sugar. He wants them to check their blood sugar three times a day, two hours after meals.

Dr. Lewis tells patients newly diagnosed with type 2 to lose weight by reducing fat and sugar and by exercising vigorously six days a week. He has them test their blood before breakfast and before and after exercise for two weeks and report to him by phone.

Dr. Day tells newly diagnosed patients with type 1 diabetes to take four insulin injections a day, do carbohydrate counting at their meals and snacks, and test their blood sugar before every shot and at bedtime.

Which of these doctors is right? It depends.

Treatment Depends on Several Factors

Treatment depends on whether the patient has type 1 or type 2 diabetes. It depends on the patient's weight. It depends on the patient's regular physical activity. It depends on what the doctor knows about the patient's resources and obligations and how they will make it easier or harder for the patient to follow certain aspects of a particular diabetes plan. It depends on what the doctor's training was and how rigorous he or she believes diabetes treatment has to be. Dr. Day, for example is an endocrinologist (gland/diabetes specialist). Endocrinologists receive years of training and practice in treating patients with diabetes so they are experienced in insulin adjustments and other fine points of diabetes management.

It depends on the latest scientific data the doctor may have read or heard at a recent medical meeting.

Nearly everything about diabetes management "depends."

Weight

The patient's weight can have an impact on what medications, activity, and diet the physician prescribes.

As you can see from the four doctors' diet instructions above, there isn't one "right" diet. Some patients only need to limit sugar and carbohydrates while others also need to reduce fat and calories.

Reducing fat and calories, in addition to carbohydrate, is especially important for most people over 40 who get diabetes. About eight out of ten of them are overweight. But if a doctor has been seeing a patient for years, and for years has been recommending without success that the patient lose weight, the doctor may give up on that area and concentrate on other changes in diet, such as reducing sweets and eating at scheduled times.

Patient Resources

A patient's resources often dictate what a physician can and can't include in a diabetes plan. When we say "resources" we usually think of financial means. But resources also cover the patient's lifestyle (which includes family help, job demands, and nearness to medical facilities), emotional health, and mental and/or physical skills that could make some aspect of the diabetes plan impractical or impossible.

Poor Vision

Some patients are very able mentally to make responsible decisions but have poor eyesight. Actually, the visually impaired and even those who are completely blind are less dependent than you might expect. There are blood sugar testing meters that "talk" and insulin-measuring devices that allow accurate dosing without the aid of a sighted human helper. However, there are two areas that the visually handicapped may not be able to manage alone: checking their feet and transportation to doctors. Your help with these might be much appreciated.

Patient Resistance

Some patients simply will not stop smoking or drinking to excess. Others won't exercise regularly, lose weight, reduce sugar, or take insulin. Perhaps they've tried to diet or stop smoking or drinking in the past, but have failed. Maybe they just aren't willing to fail again. For some people, taking insulin shots is so fear provoking that they can't bring themselves to do it. In the case of a patient with type 1 diabetes who needs insulin to survive, the fear of death eventually overcomes the fear of the needle. But in the case of a patient with type 2 diabetes whose blood sugar remains high on oral medication but who can stay alive without insulin, the threat of future complications may not be enough to make that person give himself or herself injections.

Some health professionals try lectures and threats of complications to overcome patient resistance. Others have learned that counseling and behavior modification can produce good results with most resistant patients. Often the problem is finding insurance coverage for counseling.

Learning Problems

Rigidity and fear aren't the only barriers to a patient taking care of himself or herself. Sometimes the person is not intellectually capable of learning the skills necessary to treat diabetes effectively. Learning deficiencies can prevent a person from using a blood sugar meter, following a diabetic meal plan, or accurately measuring an insulin dose. For this person, a plan may have to be simplified to "Don't eat sugary foods and don't eat a lot of food at one meal." Sometimes a visiting nurse, friend, or relative must fill insulin syringes, give injections, or test blood, at least for a time. If no dependable professional or loved one can help at home, the person may have to live in a group home where a caregiver can do the essential diabetes tasks.

Blood Sugar Testing

Testing blood sugar is a key aspect of diabetes treatment that varies tremendously according to the physician's beliefs and the patient's resources. Frequently, all the factors already mentioned influence when, where, how, and if a patient tests. Another factor is whether the patient thinks it's worth the time and money.

Testing Without Knowing Why, Is Not Enough

Blood sugar testing sometimes seems a waste of time to people who prick their fingers, do the test, fill in their logs, and show three months of tests to their doctor during an office visit, only to have the doctor barely glance at the figures. Or sometimes the doctor looks at the numbers and changes the medication dosage without telling the patient what he or she noticed that justified the change. That's a pity.

The more the physician involves the patient in the decision-making process and the better the person understands the balance of insulin, exercise, and food, and how they affect the blood sugar, the more likely he or she is to learn how to control each factor and to appreciate the importance of blood sugar tests.

Many studies have shown that blood sugar testing alone does not improve blood sugar control because the essential factor is not the testing, but the patient's *knowing what to do with the results* of the tests. If the physician or a diabetes educator can get across the idea that blood testing is a *tool for the person with diabetes*, what once was just the doctor's, nurse's, or dietitian's demand can become meaningful to the patient. Those numbers can actually help him get and keep control of his diabetes management.

When To Test

As part of the diabetes management plan, a physician recommends what times of day the patient should test. Some doctors believe that the most important blood sugar reading is the one before breakfast. That's called the fasting blood sugar because the patient has had nothing to eat all night while asleep. Food is then largely eliminated as a possible factor. The fasting levels recommended are 80-120 or 90-130 depending on which guideline is being followed.

Other doctors say that it's pretty easy to get the fasting blood sugar under control, but it's the postprandial ones (after meals) which can stay high for hours, that need to be brought to light and be dealt with. These physicians want their patients to test two hours after meals (timing starts with the first bite of food) and to have a blood sugar level under 180. If the level is higher, the patients know they ate too much at the previous meal or ate too much carbohydrate, maybe even some concentrated form they may not have known was in the food, such as honey or corn syrup. Those patients are given information about modifying their food intake.

How Often To Test

Doctors usually order more frequent blood testing if the patient is on diabetes medication, whether that is pills, insulin, or both. That's because medication lowers blood sugar, sometimes too much. By testing, a person can find out if the level is low or is likely to get too low and can eat something to correct or prevent it. Times when that is likely to happen are when the person exercises, delays or skips a meal, or eats less than usual.

How frequently the doctor orders blood testing may depend on other factors. A recent change in medication, diet, exercise, or illness usually requires closer monitoring of blood sugar, at least temporarily.

Another factor in the frequency of blood testing is the patient's previous experience: recent excessively high or low blood sugar levels may indicate that more monitoring is necessary. Some patients have stable blood sugar that varies little once they can control the portion sizes of meals. Others can adhere to a strict diet, exercise the prescribed amount, take the same dosage of medication, and still have high and low blood sugar readings seemingly without rhyme or reason. Frequent testing for these people helps them predict and prevent some of those highs and lows and may help them discover the causes. And if the cause can be discovered and eliminated, the person can test less frequently.

More frequent testing is also desirable when a person has lost some or all sensitivity to the signs of low blood sugar. Normally, low blood sugar makes a person feel sweaty, shaky, hungry, and nervous. These are signs that some food or juice is needed to raise blood sugar. Some people do not have these early warning signs. This is called hypoglycemia unawareness. It could be because they have low blood sugar often and have thereby depleted the alarm hormones that give the signal, or they may be taking a medicine that blocks these hormones. The first they may know of a low blood sugar is when a paramedic is leaning over them and they're being given glucose by vein. For them, testing whenever there is a possibility of low blood sugar, such as after exercise, is essential.

Hypoglycemia unawareness can be treated by allowing blood sugar to run a little high for a week or two by decreasing the insulin dosage. This allows the hormone levels to return to normal so the person has recognizable symptoms again.

Blood Sugar Testing and Lifestyle

A patient's lifestyle can affect how often a physician prescribes blood sugar testing. For example, a person who lives alone may need to test more frequently because there is no one around to help spot symptoms of a low blood sugar and run to get a glass of juice.

Athletes often test before, during, and after intense exercise. The "after" testing may be at intervals of several hours, even more frequently the next day. One woman in training for a triathalon felt fine all day Sunday during and after hours of running, cycling, and swimming, but collapsed from low blood sugar at her desk the next day.

Another good candidate for frequent blood sugar testing is someone who operates machinery or has some other job of special responsibility, such as caring for young children. They have to be extra careful about preventing muddled thinking, disorientation, or the worst-case scenario—a loss of consciousness—that very low blood sugar can cause.

Blood Sugar Testing and Financial Resources

Another factor in deciding how often blood testing is done is money. We hate to admit that people's health can be compromised by the dollar, but it is. Blood testing strips are about 70 cents to $1.00 each. A patient who is not taking insulin may not have insurance approval for blood testing supplies. Or the person may not have *any* insurance. Even if the patient's medical condition dictates that testing is needed four times a day, if the $70+ a month isn't there, the patient can't test as often as needed.

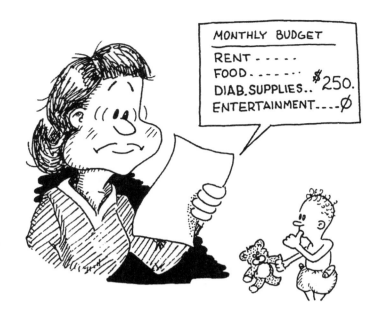

Past Experience of a Physician Influences Treatment

In addition to the strengths and limitations that the patient brings to the treatment options, the physician also has experiences that have an impact on diabetes management decisions.

For many years a debate raged in the medical community regarding the usefulness of insisting that patients try to maintain a normal blood sugar level. Many physicians, backed by the American Diabetes Association, believed that high blood sugar was responsible for the complications that people got after decades with diabetes. These doctors prescribed diabetes treatment plans designed to keep blood sugar as close to normal as possible. These more intensive regimens were a lot of work for the doctor and the patient. They required discipline and cost more. The proponents claimed that the effort paid off. But not all doctors agreed.

The dissenting physicians felt it was worth trying to prevent very high blood sugar requiring hospitalization, but that more than this was not very beneficial. They believed that complications would develop regardless of how aggressive the treatment plan was, so why burden the patient with extra work and expense?

Both groups of physicians relied on their training and experience to back up their conclusions. Until recently there wasn't a clinical study that unequivocally proved either point of view. Now there is.

What We Know Now

In June 1993 at the American Diabetes Association's annual convention, the results of the *Diabetes Control and Complications Trial (DCCT)* were presented for the first time. The statistics from this nine-year study of 1441 people with type 1 diabetes showed that the incidence and severity of complications can be significantly reduced by keeping the blood sugar level as close to normal as possible. The data that back up this conclusion include photographs of the interior of eyes and lab tests that show kidney function. These are both objective measurements of physical status, not merely opinions.

Proof of the blood sugar level was provided by another objective laboratory test, not by patients monitoring themselves on portable meters and recording the results. The blood sugar level was determined from a blood sample drawn in the doctor's office or clinic and sent to a laboratory. The labs performed a relatively new test, at that time, that reflects how often blood sugar has been high over the last three months. The glycohemoglobin, or glycosylated hemoglobin, or hemoglobin A1c test (now usually written A1c) measures the amount of glucose that has "stuck" to the hemoglobin part of red blood cells during the lifetime of the cells, and cannot be altered by anything the patient does a day or so before the blood is drawn. (Until this new test came along, patients could fast for two days before a scheduled office visit so that their blood sugar lab result would show a normal value. Of course, this made the test useless but the patient avoided a long lecture from the doctor for being in poor control.) The A1c enabled researchers to objectively compare blood sugar levels with the changes, if any, in eye and kidney health.

Advantages of Intensive Treatment

The patients in the group that had monthly medical visits and who took insulin at least three times a day (called the intensive management group) had the most normal A1c tests and had the least deterioration in their medical condition over the nine years of the study. Even patients who had already shown some damage before the study began, had a reduction in the damage by maintaining near normal blood sugars for the years of the study. Intensive therapy reduced by 45% the risk of developing vision-threatening forms of retinopathy (disease of the retina of the eye) or retinopathy requiring laser treatment. Serious kidney disease was reduced by 56%, serious nerve disease was reduced by 60%, and the risk of developing a high level of LDL (bad) cholesterol that could lead to strokes and heart attacks was also reduced.

To attain this almost normal blood sugar required a lot of extra work on the part of the patient and health care team. More frequent injections meant more frequent testing. The monthly visits with a physician or diabetes educators for any necessary adjustments of medication, diet, and other treatment elements were costly in time for both the patients and the medical team. In contrast, the group that received the standard treatment of one or two injections a day was seen four times a year by the health care team. The progression of diabetes complications in this standard therapy group was significantly higher.

So now there is *proof* that maintaining blood sugars in the normal range results in a decrease in the nerve and blood vessel damage that causes complications.

The DCCT study puts to rest the debate about whether complications are a necessary consequence of diabetes. They are not. *Complications are a result of high blood sugar.* To the extent that high blood sugar can be prevented, the incidence and severity of complications will be reduced.

After the study ended, the standard group participants largely adopted what the intensive group had been doing. The intensive participants stopped being quite as diligent. So except for nobody going to the doctor every month, they had a lot in common.

But years later there are still differences in the effects of the better blood sugar the intensive group had for the 6½ years of the study.

When the DCCT ended in 1993, researchers continued to study more than 90% of the participants. In this follow-up study, the EDIC, they found further benefits of intensive treatment including a 42% reduced risk of any cardiovascular disease event and a 57% reduced risk of nonfatal heart attack, stroke, or death from cardiovascular causes. Ten years later, those participants who were in the intensive group also continued to have significantly less eye, kidney and nerve disease.

This indicated that taking care of diabetes in the early years paid off into the future.

Disadvantages of Intensive Treatment

There is a downside to intensive treatment, however. First is the expense of taking more shots and testing more often.

Another disadvantage is the slightly increased incidence of serious, unexpected low blood sugar events. "Serious," means a low blood sugar that requires the help of another person because the person with diabetes is temporarily too impaired to get a glass of juice or eat glucose tablets. The goal of intensive treatment is to keep the blood sugar close to normal levels. That results in a smaller safety margin before it gets too low. Some people who live alone or operate machinery would not be able to safely maintain a near-normal blood sugar if they experienced surprise lows as a side effect. Although low blood sugar that needed help occurred more often in the DCCT study participants, the average was only one additional serious low blood sugar event every two years.

Doctors Weigh Several Factors Before
Recommending Intensive Treatment

Do not expect, however, that every doctor will jump to change every diabetic patient's treatment plan based on the findings of the DCCT and other research studies. Some will want more proof; some will resist because they are so convinced that what they personally see in their practices is the truth; and some will feel that the costs in time and expense to their patients, especially their elderly patients, will not pay off.

Intensive Treatment For Older and Younger Folks

There are several advantages to intensively treating older adults even if they do not have a life expectancy of an additional 50 years. First, complications can begin appearing after only five years with the disease. Further, many people who are diagnosed in their middle years or later, have already had it "silently" for several years with damage from high blood sugar already present. If we add the fact that the fastest growing age group in this country is that of people over 85, it's clear that a 65-year old newly diagnosed with diabetes may well live long enough to develop serious complications.

We know, too, that managing type 2 diabetes well also pays off. The UKPDS, a large study of over 5,000 people with type 2 showed that lowering blood sugar *and* blood pressure levels reduces the risk of heart disease, stroke, diabetic eye and kidney disease.

The strongest argument against intensive treatment for older adults is that low blood sugar can be dangerous, especially for people with hardening of the arteries. Strokes and heart attacks have been brought on by low blood sugar. However, if the patient is medically able and willing and can *safely* follow a strict treatment plan, the fact that he or she is 65 or older should not be the sole deterrent.

For children, especially those under two, intensive treatment, which attempts to keep blood sugar in the normal range, can be risky. Since low blood sugar can impair normal brain development, which is not complete until seven years of age, it is safer to allow the blood sugar to remain slightly higher until the child is older and is better able to assist in intensive diabetes management.

Patients' Patience and Doctors' Patience

Yet another factor that influences how aggressively a doctor will get with a diabetes treatment program is how discouraged the physician is by patients' resisting medical advice. Some patients may believe that doctors see them only as people with diabetes, whereas patients see themselves primarily as mothers, employers, students, and basketball fans and, second, as people who happen to have diabetes. They commonly complain that their doctors want them to measure their food, check their blood sugar too frequently, exercise every day, write everything down, and on and on. And sometimes their moms or some other important someone joins the doctor in the sermon titled "You have to take your diabetes seriously–it's important!"

And the person with diabetes says, "I know it's important, but, be real: I have a job. I have a life. I can't just do diabetes stuff all the time."

What is a doctor to do when he or she has just examined another patient who will lose a foot or whose kidneys have failed and will need dialysis, and whose next patient is one who won't follow the doctor's advice? The consequences of sloppy diabetes management are very real to that doctor. However, to the patient they may be only a remote possibility in the distant future.

Remember, most doctors chose medicine to help people. They can't help, however, if people won't come in for checkups because they think the doctor is too demanding. So maybe your friend's doctor doesn't even mention that exercise six times a week is a good idea. If the patient says she's doing it three times a week in a good week, the doctor may give up with a "Do the best you can." Many good physicians have learned to walk a narrow line between urging what they know their patients should be doing and what they know those patients are willing to do.

The bottom line, though, is that the physician also knows that if the patient does not give time and attention to the inconvenient tasks of diabetes today, he or she may well pay with a lot more than inconvenience in a few years.

Intensive or Routine: Which Treatment Plan Does Your Friend or Family Member Have?

If doctors expect different things from their patients for many different reasons, what can you assume your friend or family member has been told by their doctor? Not much. They may have a doctor who is trying to keep their blood sugar normal or one who interferes minimally with the course of diabetes. The person with diabetes may also tell you something very different from what he or she said and heard in the doctor's office.

How You Can Help Your Relative or Friend Get the Best Treatment

Learn to Ask the Right Questions

If it's your responsibility to help manage your family member's diabetes treatment, you may have to learn the right questions to ask. This requires getting the kind of information this book and others have to offer. The "Resources" in the Appendix is a good place to find out more.

At the rate that diabetes knowledge is growing, even a five year old book may be out-of-date. Don't ignore books, though. That would be like throwing the baby out with the bath water. Just don't make any *decisions on treatment* based on what could be old information. The diabetes magazines listed under "Suggested Reading" are good sources on the latest in treatment and products.

Medicine is a changing science, so trying to determine if your loved one's doctor is doing the right thing is not easy. One way you can learn what is considered basic diabetes care by the American Diabetes Association is to send for their *Standards of Medical Care for Patients with Diabetes Mellitus*. This short guide was developed by 150 medical professionals experienced in diabetes treatment. The *Standards* outline and define what the physician should ask and check during the physical exam, what tests he or she should order, how often referrals should be made to eye and other specialists, how often return visits should be scheduled, and so forth.

A phrase that medical people sometimes hear is, "That doctor orders a lot of tests just to pad the bill." Another is, "Whenever you go to the doctor, he sends you to another one. They're all in cahoots to get a lot of money."

The Standards of Medical Care not only will allow you to assure yourself that everything is being done that should be done, it also will help you and your relative or friend with diabetes understand why the doctor is recommending some tests and specialist consultations.

Certain tests are absolutely necessary to know what is happening with the kidneys, eyes, and inside blood vessels. There is simply no way to know if there is early or even moderate damage just by how he or she feels. Only a blood test, thorough eye exam, and urine test, will answer the question, "Is the treatment my dad or my sister getting the right one? Is a change needed?"

If your presence is welcome, go into the doctor's office with your family member or friend. Four ears are better than two. Take notes. Together you will remember more of the doctor's instructions and comments and will be more likely to remember to ask all the questions you thought of on the way to the doctor's office. By the way, between appointments, write down your questions and try to get them all answered before you're ushered out.

An office nurse suggested that you'll have a better chance of this happening if you ask whoever takes you both into the examining room, to pass the list on to the doctor *before* he or she comes into the room. That way if the doc needs to check anything in the records, he or she will have all the facts.

Celeste, who's had type 1 diabetes for 14 years, says, "No matter how silly you think the questions might be (they probably aren't, though), ask them, and make sure you fully understand the answers before you leave." Celeste's advice applies to you, as helper, too.

Another reason two listeners are better than one, is that sometimes the patient hears only the diagnosis. The anxiety that comes with hearing the words *insulin* or *kidney disease* can block out everything that the doctor says after that. And if the instructions sound like new information or are complicated, ask the doctor to write them down.

Increasingly, doctors print out visit summaries which include the purpose of the visit, tests needed, recommendations, new medications, etc. Aren't computers (at least occasionally) wonderful!

If the doctor recommends some treatment that your friend or family member is afraid to follow, *be sure the doctor knows this.* One example is a fear of low blood sugar if insulin is increased. *The patient should leave the office convinced of the benefits of following this recommendation (or any other) and armed with ways to prevent or handle any possible consequence.* For example, most low blood sugar episodes can be anticipated by more frequent blood glucose testing and by matching insulin to meals and exercise or vice versa.

Doctors with the best intentions may recommend changes that your family member or friend does not believe are possible. Quitting smoking, drinking, and/or losing weight are three hard changes to make and stay with. If the physician is made aware the patient probably cannot make such changes without more help, the doctor will be able to recommend a supplemental program of smoking cessation, alcohol counseling, or weight control. If your special someone has tried self-control and it hasn't worked, it's time to try "Plan B" or some more creative alternative.

New medications and changes in medication can bring new situations. For those on oral medication, a frequent question is "What should I do if I forget to take my medicine?" Depending on the dosage and the medication, the doctor may say, "Take it now, even if it's two hours late" or "Take the next dose at the usual time." This is a good question to ask before you leave the office. You can also ask about possible side effects at this time, but there is another excellent source for this information–the pharmacist.

The Pharmacist Can Help

If you pick up medication for someone, ask the pharmacist about side effects; if the medicine should be taken before, with, or after a meal; if there is a generic form that is comparable; if there's any medicine or food that is a bad combination with this medicine; if even small amounts of alcohol can cause a reaction; and if it's all right to drive after taking this medication. In fact, these are good questions to ask about any medicine—not just pills that lower blood sugar.

Many people take several medications, which may interact in unexpected ways with each other. The pharmacist can help anticipate problems with incompatible medicines. Nowadays, most pharmacies have computer files listing all customers' medications. These files can alert the pharmacist to problem combinations—*if* the customer buys all his or her medications at the same pharmacy or tells the pharmacist everything else being taken.

The Dentist and Periodontist

The same changes that occur in the blood vessels of the eyes and other organs of someone with diabetes, can occur in the gums and the bone surrounding the teeth. And the reduced ability to fight infections can result in a greater chance of having mouth infections. One way the dentist has of suspecting that diabetes is not well-controlled, is if there are several gum abscesses or bone is being lost from around the teeth.

A person who has had diabetes a long time has a greater risk of periodontal (gum) disease, the infection that destroys the bone around the teeth. It is a very common problem in most people, but it can be especially severe in someone with diabetes. It is also important to know that since gum problems are infections, they can make the management of the diabetes more difficult by raising blood sugar. So diabetes can make gum disease worse, and gum disease can make diabetes harder to control.

Some of the common signs of periodontal disease are bleeding gums, teeth that move out of position, multiple gum infections, partial dentures that don't fit well, and a bad taste or bad breath. A dentist is the person to see if you suspect a periodontal problem.

The good news is that if gums are healthy to begin with, and are *kept* that way with daily brushing and flossing and twice a year cleaning by a dental hygienist, there is no reason to believe that the person with diabetes will have more problems than the non-diabetic.

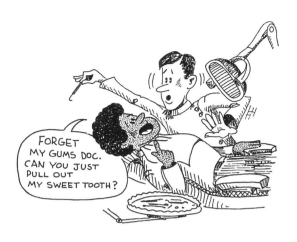

FORGET MY GUMS DOC. CAN YOU JUST PULL OUT MY SWEET TOOTH?

Other Treatment Partners

Diabetes treatment is a team effort. The person with diabetes is really the most valuable player. Nothing anyone else on the team does can do much good if the star doesn't learn and practice good management.

Other team members can help a lot, though. They include the primary care provider (physician, nurse practitioner, or physician's assistant), dietitian, nurse educator, exercise physiologist, counselor, podiatrist (foot specialist), pharmacist and ophthalmologist (eye specialist). Any of these could also be Certified Diabetes Educators (CDEs). CDEs have significant additional knowledge about diabetes management that includes diet, exercise, medications, teaching, etc. Therefore, they are able to see beyond their own specialties.

The whole team won't always be necessary, but they do have special skills your friend or family member can use from time to time.

Don't forget that you too are a member of the team. Your help can keep your relative, colleague, or friend on track. Diabetes is too complex and too changeable to be a one-man or one-woman show.

5

So Many Chores–
So Little Time

What does someone with diabetes have to do to manage this condition? A lot. Just how much "a lot" is for your friend or family member depends on several things. Most important is whether they have type 1 or type 2 diabetes.

Why The Type Of Diabetes Is Important

The type of diabetes is very important in determining the treatment plan because people with type 1 diabetes generally have more erratic blood sugars, so they need to balance food, insulin, and exercise more precisely than someone with type 2. In the past, more careful balancing required closer control of the timing and amounts of carbohydrates eaten. In the days when type 1s took only two shots a day, their lives needed to be very regimented or they risked highs and lows several times a day.

Now, they take more shots and get a more normal life. Most of them take rapid-acting insulin (Apidra, Humalog, or Novalog) before each meal and a shot of long-acting insulin (Levemir or Lantus) at bedtime. Rapid-acting insulin comes close to what insulin from a pancreas would do at mealtimes–it gets the sugar out of the blood and into the cells within 2 to 3 hours. By 3 to 4 hours it's lost most of its strength. That's good because it means there's less chance of a low blood sugar between meals. The older, slower mealtime insulins would hang around too long (up to 7 hours) making between meal snacks necessary.

People taking a rapid-acting injection before each meal do not have to eat "by the clock." In fact, a meal can be delayed, or even skipped, with less chance of going too low. Also, the content of the meal can vary much more than is possible with a longer acting insulin taken hours before. Nowadays, a person can look at their plate of food, calculate how many grams of carbohydrate (see Chapter 6) are on it, and take a dosage of insulin that will "take care of" that amount of carbohydrate.

Folks with type 2 who use insulin, don't usually need to take four shots a day because they still produce some of their own insulin. If they take insulin, they are more likely to take a long-acting insulin at bedtime. That may be enough to control their frequent high morning sugar levels. If those are normalized, they often produce enough insulin with normal activity, and with the help of diabetes pills, to get good control the rest of the day. For some type 2s their blood sugar tests make it clear that this is not working. Their doctors then might recommend two injections a day–one in the morning and one at bedtime.

These very different treatment plans involve different chores.

Chores For Those With Type 1 Who Take
Four Injections a Day

Currently, most people with type 1 diabetes are on a four injection per day routine, called an intensive insulin regimen. This is what a typical day of diabetes chores is like for 22 year old Julie:

6:15	Examine feet after shower and apply foot lotion.
6:30	Check blood sugar before taking insulin.
6:33	Write result in logbook.
6:37	Measure and inject rapid-acting insulin (dosage may vary depending on blood sugar result and amount of carbohydrate she plans to eat for breakfast so she might have to consult a chart).
6:40	Write insulin dosage taken in logbook.
7:00	Eat breakfast following prescribed meal plan. (Nothing diabetes-related until exercise or lunch.)
11:50	Check blood sugar before taking insulin and write result in logbook.
11:55	Measure and inject rapid-acting insulin (dosage may vary depending on blood sugar result and amount of carbohydrate she plans to eat for lunch so she might have to consult a chart).

11.57	Write insulin dosage taken in logbook.
12:00	Eat lunch following prescribed meal plan. (Nothing diabetes-related until exercise or dinner.)
6:00	Check blood sugar before exercising.
6:03	Write result in logbook.
6:05	Eat granola bar or 1/2 sandwich because blood sugar was low-normal and will go down more with exercise.
6:10	Play tennis (not a very strenuous or long game so no need to stop midway to check blood sugar or snack).
6:50	Check blood sugar before taking insulin.
6:53	Write result in logbook.
6:55	Measure and inject rapid-acting insulin (dosage may vary depending on blood sugar result and amount of carbohydrate she plans to eat for dinner so she might have to consult a chart).
6:58	Write insulin dose taken in logbook.
7:00	Eat dinner following prescribed meal plan.
10:30	Bedtime snack
10:35	Check blood sugar before taking insulin.
10:37	Write result in logbook.
10:40	Measure and inject long-acting insulin (dosage may vary depending on tonight's blood sugar or recent levels at other times of day so she might have to consult a chart).
10: 45	Write insulin dosage taken in logbook. (Nothing diabetes-related until morning).

This plan is basic and involved 23 diabetes-related chores, chores that wouldn't be necessary if Julie's pancreas were working. But Julie has to "think" for her pancreas and supply the insulin at the appropriate time and in the right amounts. This schedule is for a routine day for Julie, without an unusually high or low blood sugar. If she had had a high, she might have required a bigger dosage of insulin or even an extra injection. A low might have meant eating or drinking something to bring the blood sugar back to normal.

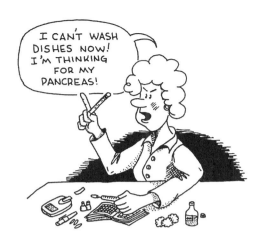

Checking Blood Sugar Levels With A Meter

An intensive insulin regimen is only possible because meters providing blood sugar readings are now available.

Nowadays there are many meters and even some new devices called continuous glucose monitors.

Meters not only measure the sugar in the blood, they remember the test results (from 10 to 3,000!), depending on the brand of meter. In addition, some meters allow entering insulin dosages, carbohydrate grams eaten at a meal or snack, give 14-day and monthly averages, and much more. This makes writing everything down in a log book redundant.

Better yet, most modern meters permit the meter to be hooked up to a computer to download and process the results, even providing graphs to show blood sugar ups and downs. Having such results might make it easier for the person with diabetes to recognize patterns of blood sugar changes.

It is also possible to rapidly send days of stored meter results over phone lines to the physician's office. There the physician or nurse specialist can assess the patterns and make changes in insulin that are more timely than was ever before possible when patients would just read off blood sugar values over the phone and all data had to be transcribed, compiled, and calculated by hand.

Not everyone finds these many features a plus. There are basic meters for people who aren't technology enthusiasts. They give blood sugar results and store them in the memory just in case you want them some day. Period. Different strokes for different folks.

The good news about doing a home blood test is that maintaining superior blood sugar levels is possible as it never was before meters.

The bad news is that the person with diabetes has to prick his finger, hand, arm, or someplace else in order to get a drop of blood to test. Fortunately, newer meters require much less blood so the puncture doesn't have to be as deep and the palm of the hand or arm (areas with fewer nerve endings), can be used.

When the new meters advertised the advantage of alternate sites, I tried them out. Whenever possible, I try to get an idea of what my patients face so I merrily did eight tests using my arm. Three of those pokes resulted in quarter-sized bruises that took three weeks to completely disappear. From my experience, anyone fair skinned might want to use the heel of the hand or stay with the fingers.

There's a tip we teach to using the fingers: generally the side of the finger-tip has fewer nerve endings than the tip or pad of the finger. Plus, one isn't hitting keyboards, etc. with that surface and feeling the tender spot again and again..

The device that makes the puncture is called a lancet. Most people load them into a adjustable, holder, which requires just the push of a button to automatically spring-propel the lancet to the correct depth.

Each brand of meter has a different procedure for getting the blood drop on the treated strip into the meter.

On the back of every meter is the company's 800-number. It is manned 24 hours a day, 7 days a week by a technician who can answer any questions about using the meter—even including walking the caller through the process of a test step-by-step. This service is free.

Experience and good blood sugar record keeping, whether by sophisticated computer process or simple pen and log book notations, tell the person and the doctor what, if any, changes need to be made in the timing, type, or dosage of medication.

Continuous Glucose Monitors

A continuous glucose monitor (CGM) does what a meter does but gives a reading every 5 minutes or less. To make this possible, the device uses a sensor with a hair-thin wire the patient inserts just beneath the skin and leaves there for 3 to 7 days (depending on the make). The sensor checks the glucose levels in tissue fluid and sends a wireless signal to a receiver which gives the glucose level and even sounds an alarm if the level is higher or lower than the range the user set.

Some people get all excited when they first hear about CGMs because they think they won't have to poke their fingers anymore. They still do, but only a couple times a day to calibrate the device. That's really a small price to pay for getting dozens and dozens of readings– even during the night.

Getting all those blood sugar readings enables doctors to adjust insulin dosages and timing much more precisely. This makes better blood sugar control possible.

Patients report they have fewer low blood sugars and less fear of going too low–two very significant benefits.

CGMs cost about $900, and the sensors run about $35-75. Insurance coverage is increasingly available.

Many people who have a CGM, also use an insulin pump. Both require being willing to learn new skills but they can lead to much improved blood glucose levels.

The Insulin Pump

There is another way of taking insulin that tries to mimic a working pancreas but that doesn't require four injections a day. That is the insulin pump. The pump is a beeper-sized computer worn on a belt or in a pocket or bra. It holds an insulin cartridge and releases a measured amount of insulin through a tube and into the body.

Don has a pump. He had to learn how to use it because it's very different from injections.

With the pump, Don attaches a piece of flexible tubing about the thickness of a strand of uncooked spaghetti and 24 to 42 inches long, depending on where he plans to insert it and how much length he needs. At the other end of the tubing, is a short, flexible hollow piece of plastic he inserts under his skin and then tapes down.
Next, he pops the insulin cartridge into the pump case, and programs the computer to give him varying doses of insulin at various times.

Don programs the pump's computer to give him a basal rate, which is half of the total amount of insulin he takes a day spread over the entire twenty-four hours. The pump gives it to him a drop at a time, which is much more like what the pancreas does.

Before a meal, Don checks his blood sugar, estimates how much he plans to eat, and programs the pump to give him a larger amount of insulin all at once, called a bolus. After the bolus is delivered, the pump returns to the basal rate and keeps giving him tiny amounts until he programs another change.

He can reduce the rate if he's going to exercise, or stop the pump if he wants to take it off to participate in contact or water sports or sexual relations. If he stays off the pump for more than two hours, he may have to take an injection to compensate for not getting insulin from the pump.

Incidentally, not everyone removes the pump when they're being amorous. One young mother told me she just lays the pump next to her in bed–she does her thing and it does its.

The pump is not something that one buys at any drugstore or orders from a catalog. Don attended a couple of support group meetings of pump users to learn if he really wanted to take on this new challenge. His doctor wrote a letter to the insurance company to explain why the pump would be a better treatment than injections for Don. His doctor also wrote that she had confidence that Don would continue to test frequently and follow the safety practices the pump requires, such as changing the tubing at least every three days.

After the insurance company approved the expense, Don started his pump education.

Because of frequent (four to eight times a day) blood glucose tests necessary to use the pump safely, it is not for someone who is "tired of doing all this diabetes stuff." While it's true that Don doesn't give himself several separate injections, he has to test more frequently, insert the needle, care for the tubing, fill the insulin reservoir, and program the pump's computer. Not a lazy way of taking insulin.

The insulin pump uses only rapid-acting insulin, which has good and bad aspects. The good news is that if the blood sugar is too high or too low, the pump can be directed to increase or decrease the amount of insulin released, and it will work quickly. Unlike intermediate or long-acting insulin which, once injected, is still being absorbed for 10-24 hours, rapid-acting insulin has a short life; if too much goes in, it quickly wears off, so it requires less snacking to correct or prevent a low. And, if more insulin is needed, a pump user just presses a few buttons on the pump. Anyone else has to get out the insulin vial, syringe, swab, and find a place to take an extra injection.

The bad aspect of the pump is also due to the rapid-acting insulin it uses. The short life of rapid-acting insulin means that if anything causes an interruption in the flow, blood sugar will quickly climb. There is no reserve of intermediate insulin taken hours before and that is still being absorbed that will, at least partly, control sugar levels.

An interruption in flow can be caused by a kink in the tubing, a clog in the needle under the skin, an infection or allergy where the needle is placed that interferes with absorption, or a battery failure. Another way pump users (or any insulin user, really) can fail to get the insulin they need, is when the insulin "fries." One young woman told me her blood sugar started going up after a trip to the beach. She gave herself a bolus of insulin. Her blood sugar continued to climb. She changed her tubing and checked her battery but the level still didn't come down. The last thing she tried was changing the insulin in the reservoir of the pump, and that worked. It turned out her insulin had gotten overheated on the blanket next to her in the sun and had become ineffective. (Insulin doesn't always have to be refrigerated but it can't be kept at over 86°F for very long.) If she had not discovered the cause of the pump problem on her own, however, she wouldn't necessarily have been in danger. She could have called her physician's office for instructions and gone back to taking her previous insulin dosage by injection until the pump problem was solved.

In all the above causes of pump failure, except for actually noticing that the needle has come out, it is the blood sugar level that will alert the user that something needs adjustment. Again, pumps are for the conscientious tester, not the poorly motivated.

Who Pays For The Insulin Pump

The pump has one other big disadvantage–it is very expensive. The pump itself costs about $5,000, and supplies (tubing, etc.) run about $120 per month. In addition, two or three outpatient training classes are usually necessary. Some insurance companies will pay 80% of the initial cost and supplies, but they usually must be convinced that it will be worth the outlay by preventing expensive hospitalizations for complications that would probably occur or get worse if the candidate did not have a pump. Convincing an insurance company of the cost-effectiveness of the pump for a particular person usually means that the physician has to write letters and make phone calls to the company spelling out the medical benefits of pump therapy to the patient and the financial benefits to the insurance company.

Although Don wanted the pump to add more flexibility to his lifestyle, he and his physician had a more serious reason that convinced the insurance company it would be cheaper to pay for a pump now than complications later. Don's last eye checkup showed some unfavorable changes in the retina of his eye. Eighteen years of diabetes were taking their toll. Don, his doctor, and the insurance company wanted to prevent progression of his eye disease. The best way of accomplishing that goal was to keep his blood sugar as close to normal as possible.

So Don got his pump, and with it a better tool to delay, and maybe prevent, complications.

An Artificial Pancreas: A Prospect for the Future

An artificial pancreas would be a combination of a CGM and an insulin pump with a computer program that would automatically adjust insulin delivery based on glucose levels.

Technology is not yet at the point where we can trust mechanical devices to do this critical task automatically. We still need the patient to do the thinking.

Let's hope this dream comes true in the near future.

Eating Can Be A Chore

Since everybody has to eat, it may not seem that meals and snacks should be counted as diabetes-related chores. The reason that they are included here is that for many people with diabetes, meals are neither flexible in amount nor optional, as they are for most of us. Consistency is the key word. Meals for those who use certain pills and certain type of insulins are scheduled, mandatory, and demand mental calculations like "Is the amount of carbohydrate in my prescribed meal plan the same as the amount of this serving?"

The necessity to eat a certain amount and to eat it on time is a considerable nuisance. Until Julie started taking four shots a day, she, and most people with type 1 diabetes I have talked with, listed it as one of the top 10 diabetes "pains in the neck." Eating on schedule meant Julie had to eat when she wasn't hungry. Or maybe she didn't want to eat because she was concentrating intensely on some interesting school or work project. No matter. She *had to* stop and eat. That also meant that she often had to carry food. Now she only has to carry some form of fast acting sugar like glucose tablets or hard candies.

Being Prepared For Every Situation

Julie's schedule may be flexible, but she still carries her insulin and meter with her. That means a kit with the following supplies:

> Rapid-acting insulin
> Long-acting insulin (in case of a sleep-over)
> Syringe(s)
> Alcohol swabs (optional)
> Meter, strips, and lancet device
> Spare lancets
> Cotton balls or tissue
> Log book and a pen to record results

And you think your handbag, backpack, or briefcase is crowded! How about adding all of the above plus emergency candy, food, or juice?

There are some space-saving devices that can help a bit with the paraphernalia load. One of these is an insulin pen that holds a cartridge of insulin in a self-contained holder and needle. It eliminates the need for a vial of insulin–the syringe and vial are all incorporated into one device. Many people with diabetes use insulin pens instead of vials and syringes. Measuring is easier and it doesn't look as intimidating to new insulin users as a hypodermic syringe that's a reminder of painful vaccinations.

Another space saver is the blood glucose meter with a memory. Many of these allow the user to do scores of blood glucose tests and recall them with the push of a button. Julie's doesn't have a way to record the dosage of insulin she gave herself, though, so she still has to write *something* down. Still, the memory means she can wait to write down the results of the day's blood sugar tests until she's at home at the kitchen table–sort of like balancing your checkbook at home when you feel like it instead of while standing at the cashier's counter after every transaction.

Some new meters have drums or discs that hold at least 10 strips *inside* the meter, dispensing with the need to carry strips separately.

The bottom line, though, is that she's got to carry stuff and it's not stuff that anybody else has to bother with. It's not a *huge* pain, but it is another irritation that having diabetes brings.

Foot Care

Foot care is important for everyone with diabetes. Feet can lose sensation when high blood sugar damages nerves. It's possible to have a deep sore, cut, or a nasty infection and not feel a twinge.

People with diabetes are urged to let their eyes tell them if there is a problem. Julie checks her feet every day after her shower. She looks for white or reddened areas, blisters, ingrown toenails, and athlete's foot. She applies lotion to her feet to keep them from getting dry and cracked because cracks can be an entry point for germs.

There are many things Julie *doesn't* do because she has diabetes. She doesn't walk around barefoot or in open-toed shoes or sandals, and she doesn't use corn plasters or chemicals to dissolve corns or calluses. She certainly doesn't do "bathroom surgery" such as using razor blades to remove corns; a podiatrist does that for her.

One more thing Julie *doesn't* do is soak her feet. People used to think a nice, long soak in Epsom salts was good for feet. Well, it isn't good for diabetic feet! There are several reasons for this:

First, with poor nerve sensation, too many people have burned themselves in water that was really too hot but felt just fine to them. Even if Julie avoids that danger by using a thermometer, there's another problem.

Second, although her feet would *feel* moisturized when she pulled them out of the water, soaking is actually drying. Soaking removes the natural oils that no amount of lotion can totally replace, thereby making her skin drier and more prone to cracks and infections than before.

The last reason why soaking is not advised is that warmth to a body part increases the metabolism of the cells in that area. Usually that is not a problem. The blood vessels in the area dilate and more blood comes in with the additional food and oxygen required by the increased metabolism. But what if the blood vessels are narrowed by fatty deposits or rigid walls? In that case, the extra blood won't be able to get to the cells and they will suffer from insufficient oxygen and glucose. Some cells will even die. Hot soaks, hot water bottles, and hot pads on the feet should be avoided by people with diabetes.

So don't buy electric foot soakers as a present for someone with diabetes. Offer a gentle foot massage with lotion. We all like massages.

You may be able to help with some aspects of foot care if you live with a person with diabetes. If they have poor vision or are not very flexible and can't see all parts of their feet you could be the "foot checker."

If you go with the diabetic to the doctor's office, remind him or her to take off shoes and socks before the doctor comes in. Busy physicians can forget feet when they are checking heart, lungs, and blood pressure. Exposed feet get their attention.

Pills For Type 1 and Type 2

There are pills that people with diabetes often take that don't lower blood sugar. They are prescribed to reduce the risk of common complications. The three that most adults take are aspirin, a pill to reduce cholesterol, and a pill to help protect the kidneys.

The low-dose aspirin (usually 75-81 mg) is taken to "thin the blood" (keep blood platelets from sticking together). Someone who is taking a powerful blood thinner such as coumadin should not take aspirin. It is also not recommended in someone with a history of stomach bleeding.

A cholesterol-lowering pill (usually a statin drug) is prescribed primarily to lower LDL cholesterol but also has an additional benefit–it has an anti-inflammatory effect on blood vessels which reduces the chances of a plaque deposit breaking free.

Both aspirin and cholesterol-lowering medicines help in reducing the risk of cardiovascular diseases, the most serious complications of diabetes.

The medicines that help protect the kidneys (ACE inhibitors and ARBs) are actually mild blood pressure pills that delay the onset and progression of kidney disease. They can also reduce other complications of diabetes such as foot ulcers and eye damage.

These medicines are often prescribed for people *before* they have problems with blood clotting, cholesterol and blood pressure because of their other important actions.

Type 2 Diabetes

Some people with diabetes still have some functioning insulin-producing cells and do not need insulin as part of their treatment.

For these people, exercise and diet alone may maintain blood sugar within normal limits. For some, oral medication that lowers blood sugar may also be needed.

Oral Diabetes Medication

Oral diabetes medications are *not* pill forms of insulin. They are not effective if the cells in the pancreas no longer produce insulin. Although these drugs can't replace insulin, and are unlikely to be effective if the diet is ignored, they do have one or more of these helpful effects:

1. They stimulate the pancreas to release insulin.
2. They help insulin bind to the cell so glucose can enter.
3. They may suppress the release of glucose from the liver.
4. They may slow down the absorption of carbohydrate from the digestive system.

The result is that more insulin is available or is more effective, so more sugar is able to leave the blood and get into the cells. That means the blood sugar will go down, and without attention, it could go down too far (see Chapter 4 for more on pills).

Preventing Blood Sugar From Going Too Low

Low blood sugar can be dangerous or even fatal, so a person who is taking blood sugar lowering pills has to take some precautions, just as insulin users do. They are less likely to have a serious low blood sugar than someone using insulin, but the chance is still there.

Precautions to prevent low blood sugar include:

Not drinking alcoholic drinks without a meal
(see Chapter 9);
Not eating later than usual;
Not skipping meals;
Not eating less than the amount calculated by the physician or dietitian to match the effect of the medicine.

These precautions mean that eating on schedule is important for those on some oral medications. The low blood sugar that can occur as a consequence of not eating enough can be severe and prolonged. The severity varies with the person's condition and time without food. Most pills are meant to be effective for 12 to 24 hours, so a low blood sugar level can last a long time.

Checking Blood Sugar

Because people who take oral medication have some insulin production and a less impaired ability to regulate their blood sugar, they tend to have less erratic swings in blood sugar levels than someone who is dependent on injected insulin. This means it is usually not necessary for them to check their blood sugar as often as those with type 1 do.

Physicians have many different opinions about when and how often blood sugar needs to be checked by someone with type 2 who does not require insulin. Recommendations range from twice a week to four times a day. Some doctors ask their patients to check once a day before breakfast. Others have them check before breakfast and dinner when they usually take their pills. While some patients are learning to balance their exercise, diet, and medication, they may need to test as often as a person taking insulin. Or they may be told to test two hours *after the first bite of a meal* to check what affect the foods they just ate had on their blood sugar level. Some patients find they have very stable blood glucose levels when they stay on their diet, exercise, and medication programs, so their doctors recommend decreasing how often they check. Unfortunately, sometimes the deciding factor in how often blood sugar testing is performed is the cost of the strips, not medical necessity.

Checking Blood Sugar: The Chore Everyone Loves To Hate

Blood sugar testing is in first place of the most dreaded daily chore on everyone's list.

Reason #1: It Requires Planning and Record Keeping

Testing blood sugar requires having a supply of lancets and blood glucose strips, calibrating the blood glucose meter that reads the strips, doing periodic control solution tests, and carrying strips, meter, lancets, and a log book and pen to record the results.

Reason #2: It's Expensive

Buying the supplies is no small sacrifice for many people. Blood glucose test strips alone cost 70 cents to 1.00 each. For a person who tests four times a day, that's about $80-$120 dollars a month. Some insurance companies pay a part or all of this expense; others don't. From my own informal surveys, people have told me their basic supplies and diabetes medicine run from $30 to well over $200 a month. (Note, that this does not include any doctor fees, lab tests, or hospital bills.)

Reason #3: It's Inconvenient And Awkward

Since blood sugar testing is most often done before meals, sometimes it needs to be done in a restaurant. Some people test in their cars before going inside. Others lay out all their paraphernalia on the restaurant table, stab their finger, put the drop on the strip, and so forth–maybe while everyone else in the party is ordering. Some go to the restroom and hope there's more than a sink ledge to perch their equipment on. It depends on the restaurant and the group of diners and how comfortable onlookers are with the procedure.

Finding a clean, private nook for taking an insulin injection can also be a challenge. (That's probably why some brave souls experimented and discovered that they could inject *through* their clothing!)

Reason #4: It Hurts

Blood sugar testing generally hurts more than insulin injections because the lancet is thicker *and* there are more nerve endings in fingertips than in most injections sites. Sometimes the pain is over in a minute. Sometimes the finger is tender for hours. And when your friend or relative has 28 or more little punctures in her fingers at the end of every week, she doesn't feel much like doing the testing that makes the pricking necessary. But she does it anyway.

Reason #5: It's Something They Say I Have To Do *and* They Expect Perfection

Doctors, diabetes educators, mothers, and others tell people with diabetes to do blood sugar testing regularly. Worse, they are not always understanding about any gaps in testing or undesirable results. One 53-year old woman says her mother still grills her about her blood sugar. If it's high, she's accused of having eaten candy; if she denies it, she's called a liar.

Blood sugar seems to be the last unrespected area of privacy to many people with diabetes.

Reason #6: It's Frustrating

Imagine having stayed on your diet, exercised as you were supposed to, and taken your medicine on time but when you checked your blood sugar it was double or triple the normal level. For some, that happens often. One young woman told me that testing her blood sugar was like getting graded—with the chance of failing at every test. Add the mistaken idea of parents and others that blood sugar is perfectly controllable with diet and medicine, and you have two good reasons for frustration. It *can't* be controlled perfectly but everybody without diabetes thinks it can. This frustration, together with some people's judgmental attitude, makes infrequent testing and made-up numbers very tempting.

The mind set that views blood sugar readings not as results that are high, low or normal but as grades or moral judgments, makes blood sugar testing less likely to be done. The blood sugar level then becomes "bad" or "good," and by extension, the person whose blood gave that result is "bad" or "good."

If everyone considered blood sugar testing as merely collecting information instead of a pat on the back or a kick in the rear from on high, feeling bad could be usefully replaced by decision-making.

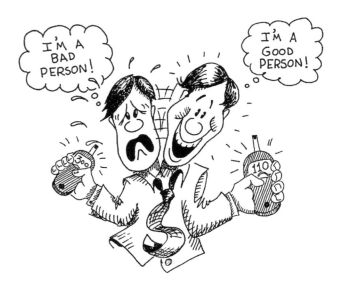

Reason #7: If I Know What My Blood Sugar Is, I'll Have To Do Something About It

Doctors tell people with diabetes to check their blood sugar regularly so they'll know when it's high or low. But lots of times your loved one or friend with diabetes doesn't want to know. If he knows, he'll have to do something about it. That something may be injecting an extra dose of insulin, eating when he's not hungry, not eating when he is, not running with the team because his blood sugar is too high, or delaying the tennis game because he has to eat a snack first. At the very least, the blood sugar level will be in his meter's memory and could bring criticism and a lecture on improving blood sugar control at his next visit to the doctor.

Chores For Someone With Type 2 Diabetes

Chores of the person with type 2 include a variety of things they might or might not need to do. Here are the recommended chores for good diabetes management of type 2 diabetes:

1. Exercise 3 to 7 times a week. (6 or 7 is best)
2. Check feet daily.
3. Limit sugary treats.

4. Lose weight or maintain ideal body weight.
5. Test blood sugar 2 to 28 times a week.
6. Eat meals on time in required amounts.
7. Take oral medication (maybe).
8. Take insulin (maybe).

The good news about type 2 diabetes is that blood sugar control is not as difficult as with type 1. Usually diet and testing are less rigorous and insulin is a "maybe," not a requirement.

The bad news is that if type 2 diabetes is not taken seriously, if the recommended chores are not done, the same complications that can happen to someone with type 1 diabetes, can happen to someone with type 2.

Shared Attitudes About Chores With Both Types of Diabetes

The chores of diabetes are many. Here's what it adds up to after 20 years for someone taking only two shots a day, checking blood glucose three times a day, exercising and checking feet once a day, seeing the doctor who takes care of their diabetes every three months, an eye doctor once a year, and reading one diabetes magazine once a month:

Diabetes magazine	240 issues
Eye doctor	20 visits
Diabetes doctor	80 visits
Exercise	7300 times
Foot checks	7300 times
Blood sugar	21,900 tests
Insulin	14,600 shots

And the chores never end. Neither can they safely be put aside like the ironing or washing the car until the person "feels like it."

Not everyone with diabetes sees the chores as a terrible burden. Some have accepted them as a normal part of their lives like brushing and flossing their teeth. My hat is off to them.

For your friend, family member, or colleague, it may not be possible yet to take these chores in stride. They may see them as painful and inconvenient reminders of their diabetes and its scary complications.

You can help by listening to the gripes. It *isn't* fair that they have diabetes to deal with every day. Eventually, they may share Celeste's (who has been living with type 1 for 14 years) attitude. She says, "I have a lot to be thankful for, and take things a day at a time so that I know my future will be the best I can make it."

6

The Diabetes Diet:
More Than Just No Sugar

Why do some people with diabetes carry snacks?
Why do some people with diabetes avoid only sugar
    while others also limit fat or protein or all three?
What is carbohydrate counting you've heard some of
    them refer to?
What kind of desserts can a person with diabetes eat?

If you share time with someone with diabetes, chances are you've wondered about these questions. This chapter gives you the answers and the basic information to understand the answers. We discuss what a person with diabetes needs to learn about food in order to follow a diabetic diet and how they and their dietitians or physicians adapt such a diet to the person's medical needs.

You'll probably be surprised at how little difference there is in the foods that are good for you and the foods that are good for a person with diabetes.

Sugar Has Its Place

Many folks believe that people with diabetes are allergic to sugar, that they should never eat it, and some even think that eating too much sugar is what caused diabetes in the first place. But eating too much sugar doesn't cause diabetes, and sugar doesn't have to be avoided completely.

Further, as discussed in Chapter 9, sugar is taken deliberately *as medicine* to normalize a blood sugar that is too low.

Having said that, eating lots of sugar-sweetened foods is discouraged because table sugar has no nutritional value and is a highly concentrated carbohydrate (3 teaspoons has the same amount of carbohydrate as 3 cups of popcorn). As you'll see later in this chapter, there is a sensible "budget" amount of carbohydrate that one ought to eat at a meal and if most of it is table sugar, there's little or no budget left for carbohydrate-containing foods with vitamins, minerals, fiber, etc.

What Foods Turn Into Sugar

Our cells need food in the form of a particular sugar called glucose and our body changes foods of all different kinds into that sugar.

About 90% of carbohydrate foods like bread and cereal is converted into glucose; about 30 to 60% of protein foods like meat, dairy foods and eggs is turned into glucose (although the process is slower than the conversion of carbohydrates), and less than 10% of fat, such as oils and the fat in meat, cheese, etc. becomes glucose. Since carbohydrates change almost completely and fairly quickly into sugar, the more carbohydrate a food contains, the more it will contribute to raising blood sugar soon after it is eaten.

So, you may think that carbohydrate foods should be avoided, and that only proteins and fats should be eaten. In fact, avoiding carbohydrates was the only "treatment" for diabetes before the discovery of insulin. That kind of diet prolonged life for people with no other options. But with today's medicines it is neither necessary nor desirable for people with diabetes to eat an unbalanced diet with only eggs, meat and certain very low carbohydrate vegetables such as cabbage and celery.

Carbohydrates Are Necessary

Typically, our bodies need a minimum of 130 grams a day of carbohydrates and the sugar they turn into for fuel (especially for the brain and nerves), and provided they're eaten in the right amounts at the right times, they are essential nutrients even for people with diabetes. In fact, about 50% of our calories should come from starchy or sweet foods like cereal, potatoes, bread, and fruit.

Protein Is Not The Perfect Food

Protein is needed to build and repair tissues, but it has been so overemphasized that many people eat more than they need, sometimes at the expense of other nutrients that are equally important. In fact, many Americans eat at least twice the amount of protein they require. This wasn't always true. At one time, many Americans lived on corn or rice; and really didn't have enough protein foods such as meat. Nowadays, with relatively cheap meat, cheese, milk and eggs, the balance has shifted.

But more serious than eating too much meat and dairy products and not enough of something else, is the strain that eating a lot of protein can put on the kidneys. People who have had diabetes for more than 15 years may begin to show kidney damage caused by years of high blood sugar and high blood pressure. Cutting back on protein for these people can slow down further damage and delay or even prevent the need for kidney dialysis or a transplant. Too much protein also increases the risk for gout, kidney stones, and osteoporosis.

Lastly, most protein foods come with a sizeable amount of fat.

Too Much Fat Is Too Darn Common

Too much fat is a problem for most of us, but it is more serious for people with diabetes because of their greater risk for clogged blood vessels, which can result in strokes, gangrene, and heart attacks. Foods high in saturated fat are of special concern since they are the ones generally believed to cause clogged blood vessels by raising cholesterol in the blood. Here's a list of some of the foods that are high in saturated fats and cholesterol:

Beef	Hot dogs	Some lunch meat	Butter
Lamb	Hamburgers	Most cheeses	Eggs
Pork	Sausages	Whole & 2% milk	Ice cream

Also any food that says on the label that it contains *hydrogenated* oils should be limited, or, better still, avoided. That's because when vegetable oils are hydrogenated (to make margarine and solid shortening, for example) they become especially harmful trans fats. Trans fats raise bad cholesterol and lower good cholesterol, a double whammy for people with diabetes since they are at higher risk for heart disease. Foods that may have hydrogenated oils include: most baked goods and mixes, processed foods such as chips, whipped toppings, etc. and anything fried in most restaurants.

In the grocery store look for "hydrogenated oil" *in the ingredient list*. Put that product back on the shelf, even if it says, "zero trans fat" on the package or nutritional label. The FDA allows up to 0.49 grams per serving of trans fat to be labeled "zero."

Since there is no safe amount of trans fat, "zero" is taken much more seriously in many European countries. For example, since 2004 in Denmark, no products with hydrogenated oil can be sold.

If you don't want to bother reading the small print on ingredient lists, buy an organic product. Hydrogenation of oils is not allowed in organic foods so there, zero really means zero.

Fats in foods are not the only concern. Calories from *any* source that we eat beyond what we immediately need are stored in the body—much of it as body fat. Since most of us in the industrialized countries are not at risk of starving, we don't need a lot of stored fat.

Fat is singled out as the food component we most need to limit, partly because it has more than twice as many calories as the same amount of protein or carbohydrate. It doesn't take much fat in addition to our carbohydrate and protein needs to put us over the number of calories we need and cause us to store it as flab.

Calories in one gram of :	
Fat	9
Carbohydrate	4
Protein	4

Still, no matter what that extra stored body fat started out as, it contributes to poor blood sugar control. This is especially true of people who get diabetes in later years—they are very often over-weight. That extra padding interferes with insulin's function, so the body needs more insulin than the pancreas can produce. That's the insulin resistance that is so common to type 2 diabetes. The result? Sugar accumulates in the blood and blood sugar goes up. Those who can lose their extra body fat can sometimes stop taking insulin or pills because the need for extra insulin is reduced.

A Body Shape That Is Especially At Risk

Where a person carries that excess fat can be as important as having extra fat to carry. The apple-shaped person is at greater risk for cardiovascular disease than the pear-shaped person. (Apple-shaped refers to those whose fat is predominantly carried above and around the waist; pear-shaped, predominantly below the waist.) Those who are shaped more like an apple have more metabolically active fat that is more easily deposited on the inside of arteries.

The pear-shaped person is at less risk for a heart attack or a stroke. It seems that excess fat around the thighs and below the waist is not the same kind that is in arteries.

Not that being voluptuously pear-shaped is *healthy,* it's just not as *unhealthy.*

What if you're not sure which body-type you or your family member, friend or colleague is? All you need is a tape measure to find out. Measure the waist.

Waist measurements that increase heart disease risk:
Most men - 40 inches or more
Most women - 35 inches or more
For Asian men - 34 inches or more
Asian women - 31 inches or more

Carbohydrate Counting

Because blood sugar rises when people eat carbohydrate, limiting the amount of carbohydrate eaten at any one time can help control how high the level rises and how long it stays high.

The carbohydrate counting, or "carb counting" system was developed to simplify meal planning for people with diabetes. In this system, foods with similar carbohydrate, fat, protein, and calorie amounts are grouped together.

Each food in the list is called a "choice." The foods in the list below each have about 15 grams carbohydrate. As you can see, the amount (1/2 cup or 1 slice) of each food in the list varies in order to keep the carbohydrate consistent.

For example, on a list of carbohydrate choices, you'd see:

1 slice bread or small roll	1 cup milk
1/3 cup pasta or rice	1/3 to 1/2 cup fruit juice
1/2 cup cooked oatmeal	1/2 banana
3 cups plain, unbuttered popcorn	12-15 grapes or cherries
1/2 cup peas, corn, or potatoes	6 chicken nuggets
1/2 cup casserole	1 Tbsp. syrup, jam, jelly, sugar, or honey

Many people are surprised at how small most of the amounts are. That's because they are amounts with 15 grams carbohydrate–not necessarily the serving size on food packages or what we're accustomed to thinking of as a serving. Some foods, like a slice of bread or 3 cups popcorn, happen to be what we might think of as servings or portions. Others, such as 1/3 cup rice or 1/2 cup casserole, are not what most of us consider a serving of rice or casserole. They are each 1 choice because each has 15 grams carbohydrate. *They are like building blocks to create an entire meal.*

The good news is that a sensible amount for most people with diabetes is 30 to 60 grams carbohydrate per meal which equals 2 to 4 carbohydrate choices so the person with diabetes can use up 2, 3, or even 4 of their choices to get a bigger amount of a given food.

Remember, foods in the same group have different amounts to keep the number of grams of carbohydrate the same. For example,

---

A sensible amount of carbohydrate for most people with diabetes is:
> Per meal: 30 to 60 grams *or* 2 to 4 choices
> Per snack: 15 to 30 grams *or* 1 to 2 choices

---

a normal serving of most cold cereals is 3/4 cup. A choice of Grapenuts, however, is only 3 tablespoons, while a choice of puffed rice is 1½ cups. One cereal can be substituted for another, but the serving size may well need to be adjusted.

The list of choices suggests many other possible trade-offs. The same 3 tablespoons of Grapenuts can be exchanged for ¼-½ bagel or 1 slice of whole-wheat toast, or a 6-inch tortilla.

Also, someone could "spend" all their 45 carbohydrate grams on a rather large baked potato. Or he could have a slice of bread, ½ cup peas, and 12 cherries for the same amount of carbohydrate.

You're probably surprised to see some of the foods in what seem to be the wrong group. For example, although we think of peas as a vegetable, they actually have so much carbohydrate in them that they are, as far as their carbohydrate content is concerned, closer to bread than they are to tomatoes, cucumbers, and broccoli. So within the carbohydrate group, starchy vegetables such as peas and corn are separated from vegetables with little carbohydrate such as broccoli and cucumbers.

Carbohydrate counting is easier when a food has a label. Look at the serving size and then at the number of grams of total carbohydrate on the label. For example, a label may give a serving size of 1 cup and the total carbohydrate as 40 grams. That's pretty clear if you want exactly 1 cup. But *if you change the serving size, you have to recalculate the amount of carbohydrate up or down.*

To complicate things a bit more, we don't always eat a food that's only carbohydrate or only protein. Even bread is a mixture of carbohydrate and protein and we eat many dishes like pizza and casseroles that have ingredients from more than one list of choices. Foods like pizza are called combination foods. In diabetes nutrition guides some popular combination foods have the number of starch, fat and protein grams itemized so that choices can be figured without too much effort.

Surprisingly, we shouldn't pay any attention to the grams of sugar listed under total carbohydrate on the label. Let me repeat that. **Ignore the sugar grams on the label**. The sugar is already included in the amount of total carbohydrate. If you only look at the sugar grams, you might be underestimating the amount of carbohydrate in that food. With the exception of some of the fiber (more about fiber later), *all of the carbohydrate turns into sugar* so the total amount of carbohydrate is what's important.

On the other hand, if you get scared off by any sugar, you'll be avoiding some foods that can be a healthy part of a meal plan. For example, a glass of milk has 12 grams of sugar. Who put it there? The cow did–it's lactose–a naturally occurring sugar. P.S. Don't think you can get around the cow by choosing lactose-free milk. Milk labeled lactose-free just has an enzyme added that splits the lactose molecule into two other sugars so it's safe for lactose intolerant folks. It doesn't decrease the amount of sugar (carbohydrate).

Calculating a Diabetic Meal Plan (formerly "Diabetic Diet")

When Anthony, a 62-year old overweight office manager, was told he had type 2 diabetes and needed to follow a diet, he expected to be handed a printed sheet with some menus on it. That's what had happened to a friend of his. Anthony was afraid he wouldn't do any better than his friend did on the printed diet–it had almost nothing on it his friend liked and was so boring that he ate more that *wasn't* on the diet sheet than *was*. A couple of weeks of that diet, and his friend had higher blood sugars than before he tried it.

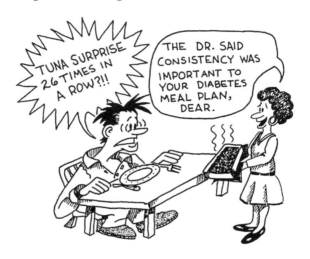

Fortunately for Anthony, his doctor sent him to a registered dietitian (RD). This is someone who has completed college and postgraduate training in nutrition and has passed a national qualifying exam. Anthony's dietitian was also a certified diabetes educator (CDE) which meant she had considerable experience counseling people with diabetes and had passed a comprehensive exam in diabetes in addition to what her RD credential required.

The dietitian made a meal plan that took into consideration Anthony's nutrition needs, how physically active he is, his schedule, and his food preferences. She also considered his doctor's recommendations (lose weight and no insulin or oral diabetes medication until diet and exercise have been given a chance to work).

The Interview with the Dietitian

The dietitian first asked Anthony's height, which was 6'1". From his height, age, body build (medium), and sedentary lifestyle, the dietitian calculated a sensible weight for him (185 pounds) and from that reasoned that a 1,600-calorie diet would be a good starting point. That may seem like a small number of calories for a man who is 6'1", but Anthony had a sedentary job and needed to lose weight to get his blood sugar under control. If he added exercise, he could eat more *or* he could exercise *and* stick with 1600 calories and get down to his goal weight more quickly.

The dietitian then used 1,600 calories to calculate how many calories of carbohydrate, protein and fat Anthony should eat every day. She then translated calories into grams and, finally, into choices.

At this point the dietitian got creative. She asked Anthony a number of questions about his meals. Did he like milk? If so, was he willing to switch from 2% milk to 1% milk? (He was.) Did he feel meat at lunch and dinner were musts? (Yes he certainly did.) Was bread and butter or margarine a staple for him at every meal? (No.) Did he usually have a snack before bedtime? (Yes.)

Based on Anthony's answers, the dietitian tailored the choices to match his preferences. For example, he said he wanted meat for lunch and dinner. Even lean meat has some fat, and since Anthony had only 50 grams of fat allotted for the whole day, some careful choosing had to be done. She left out some of the cheese, butter or margarine, and whole milk she might have included for other clients but included enough fat and protein choices at lunch and dinner so that Anthony could pick lean meat from the list of choices. Finally, she tried to spread them fairly evenly so that he got some carbohydrate, protein and fat at each meal.

There are three parts to a diabetic eating plan:

1. Type of Food
2. Portion Sizes
3. Timing

Type of Food:
Personal Preferences Are Important

Anthony's dietitian considers her clients' personal preferences and schedules very important to her clients' achieving their desired goals. She always inquires into her clients' likes and dislikes for milk, eggs, meat and other foods because most needs can be accommodated by making choices that still supply the desired amount of protein, carbohydrate and fat.

For example, some people hate skim milk and would rather have bread without butter or a bagel without cream cheese than give up their whole or 2% fat milk. Others want their red meat (even if it is only a little 3-ounce piece) rather than twice as much shrimp.

A meal plan should reflect a person's taste or it probably won't be followed.

What the dietitian came up with for Anthony was the following daily total:

Carbohydrate	12 to 15 choices
7-9 starch or bread type choices	
3-4 fruit choices	
2 cups 1% milk	
Protein/meat servings (2-3 oz each)	2
Fat choices (1 = 5 grams fat, 45 calories)	3

The dietitian then distributed the various servings among three main meals and a bedtime snack:

Breakfast		Lunch	
Carbohydrate		Carbohydrate	
Starch	2	Starch	2
Fruit	1	Fruit	1
Milk	1	Vegetables (non-starchy)	2
Protein/meat	0-1 oz	Protein/meat	2-3 oz

Dinner		Bedtime snack
Carbohydrate		Carbohydrate
Starch	3	1 starch *or*
Fruit	1	1 fruit *or*
Vegetables (non-starchy)	2	1 milk
Protein/meat	2-3 oz.	

Anthony's dietitian explained the disadvantages of eating foods high in fat (especially saturated and trans fats) and cholesterol. People with diabetes are prone to having high cholesterol and other blood fats (triglycerides are an example).

Here are Anthony's blood fat levels and the levels that would lessen his risk for a heart attack and stroke.

	Anthony's Blood Fats	**Recommended Blood Fats**
Triglycerides	415	**Under 150**
HDL cholesterol	30	**Over 40**
LDL cholesterol	220	**Under100 (or even under 70)**
Total cholesterol	250	**Under 200**

Anthony's blood fat results (plus his slightly elevated blood pressure, excess weight, and diabetes) mean that he is at moderate to high risk for a heart attack or stroke within the next 10 years. The risk comes partly from the accumulation of cholesterol deposits (plaque) on the inner walls of blood vessels; this plaque damages the vessel walls, reduces blood flow, and can break off causing a serious blockage in an artery in the heart, brain, or lungs.

Cholesterol is carried through the blood by proteins called lipoproteins. "Good" high-density lipoproteins (HDL) remove cholesterol from blood vessels and protect against heart disease.

"Bad" low-density lipoproteins (LDL) carry cholesterol from the liver, where it is made, to the blood, where it may get deposited if there is not enough HDL to remove it. (One way to remember which is which is that in school a *high* grade is *good* and a *low* grade is *bad*).

It may seem from this explanation that cholesterol is just a troublemaker, but the liver produces it for some very good reasons. Cholesterol is an important component of bile acids (important for digestion), sex hormones, vitamin D, and hormones of the adrenal gland, such as cortisone.

Useful as cholesterol may be, Anthony has too much of it. He can reduce it by eating fewer foods such as egg yolks, high fat dairy products and high fat meats that are full of saturated fats, which the liver uses to make cholesterol. Adding soluble fiber in the form of apples, oat bran, beans, etc. can also reduce cholesterol. By exercising, he can increase the level of his good cholesterol which removes cholesterol in arteries. If those three strategies don't do enough, he can also take cholesterol-lowering medication.

Most saturated fats come from animal products (meat and dairy products). Another source is the fat in margarine and shortening that starts out as unsaturated vegetable oil but is made saturated by adding hydrogen molecules. A third source is palm and coconut oil, which are saturated even without adding hydrogen.

The dietitian showed him the fat choices she included on his meal plan and explained the importance of limiting himself to two or three a day. She verified that he knew what foods to avoid or to eat only in small amounts. They reviewed the differences between the different oils.

Polyunsaturated oils (corn, safflower and sunflower) are believed to lower cholesterol levels. Monosaturated oils (olive, canola, and peanut) may also do so but their effect is less certain. Either is preferable to saturated fats, but all three have lots of calories (120 to 130 calories per tablespoon), so they should be used sparingly.

Percentage of Calories from Fat

A helpful way to become more aware of how much and what kinds of fat is in a food, is to look for total fat and saturated fat on the Nutrition Facts label. Anthony's dietitian taught him how to look at a label and calculate the percentage of fat. This is the formula:

1. Multiply the grams of fat per serving by 9. (There are 9 calories in a gram of fat).
2. Divide that number by the number of calories in a serving.
3. Multiply this number by 100.
4. The result is the percentage of fat calories in that food.

A sensible guideline is almost always to limit foods to those that are under 30% fat. Although it's true that some foods such as bread, have little or no fat, others, such as salad dressing, that are much higher in fat, can wipe out the benefit of the low fat foods in a hurry. That's why low fat salad dressings are such a help. Cookies and pastries are less likely to have low fat versions so you can assume they are usually very high in fat. For example:

Glazed doughnuts	47% fat
Lorna Doone shortbread cookie	45% fat
Bear claw pastry	54% fat

One of Anthony's earlier habits that added lots of saturated fat to his diet and contributed to his weight gain was helping himself to a Danish or two every morning at the office. His company supplies these pastries as a favor to the staff, but they're no favor to Anthony.

The dietitian explored with Anthony how best to deal with this temptation. He could ask that the pastries be stopped, thereby risking being labeled a bad guy by his co-workers. Plan number two was asking that in addition to pastries, fresh fruit be provided. That could result in unhappy management. His third option was to bring fruit or yogurt from home and eat that instead of a Danish. (Incidentally, if you have a colleague with diabetes, please back him up if he suggests healthier snacks, or propose them yourself.)

Another problem for Anthony is the frequent office birthday parties and other events with cake and cookies. He came up with a plan on his own. He decided he would take only a sliver of cake or one cookie and then stand as far away from the "temptation table" as possible.

The Good News

Not everything is a no-no. The dietitian tried to show Anthony that he doesn't have to avoid everything. She encouraged him to eat lots of vegetables and whole grains for the vitamins, minerals, and fiber they provide–not only because fiber can lower blood sugar, but also because foods with fiber tend to be more filling.

She also urged Anthony to get his fruit choices by eating whole fruit instead of by drinking juice. She explained that he would be able to eat a larger, more satisfying portion of whole fruit, plus get more healthy fiber for fewer calories.

And, of course, she explained what foods contain concentrated forms of sugar and how to substitute other foods or sweeteners. (More about sugar substitutes later in this chapter and in Chapter 7.)

When Anthony left the dietitian's office with his first meal plan, that was not the end of his instruction on diet. Most dietitians ask clients to write out several menus of their preferred foods, using the choices allotted for each meal. The client brings his menus back in a few days so the dietitian can see if he understands the plan and if it works for him. For example, if Anthony reported he felt very hungry in the afternoon, the dietitian might increase his lunch choices or add a snack even if it meant going over the original calorie limit. If Anthony ate 100 to 200 calories more a day, he could still lower his blood sugar and lose weight; it just would take longer to get to his weight goal of 185.

That kind of "fiddling" is helpful in tailoring a meal plan to the person and makes it more likely that he will be able to be successful with the new changes.

Here is a sample dinner Anthony wrote out that fits in with his 1600-calories-a-day meal plan using the dietitian's guidelines:

What the Dietitian wrote for a meal plan:	**What Anthony chose from the lists:**
1 meat serving	*3 ounces baked chicken*
4 carbohydrate choices	*1 cup boiled potatoes* (2 choices) *1/2 cup broccoli* (free) *1 small dinner roll* (1 choice) *1 lettuce-wedge salad* (free) *1 cup fresh strawberries* (1 choice)
1 fat choice	*1 Tbsp. French dressing* (1 choice)
Free beverage	*black coffee with artificial sweetener* (free)

Fortunately, there are some foods such as diet soda, coffee, bouillon, dill pickles, and lettuce that are considered "free foods" and which can be eaten at any time without measuring or exchanging. Also, most vegetables except for starchy varieties (corn, peas, potatoes, cooked dried beans, and winter squash) have so little carbohydrate per choice (5 grams) that they don't need to be counted by most peoples with diabetes.

Counting carbs and other choices may sound cumbersome, but people who use this system get very adept at looking at a plate of food and making a good educated guess as to the number of carbohydrate, meat, or other choices that are there, what they should eat, and what they should leave so they don't overshoot their meal plan.

So no fair nagging people with diabetes to clean up their plates!

Another Diabetic Meal Planning Method

Carb counting is not the only meal planning technique recommended for people with diabetes.

For some people newly diagnosed with diabetes, counting carbs, trying to understand grams and choices is overwhelming, especially with all the other diabetes recommendations they're given.

The plate method doesn't require any math or calorie counting. It relies on getting sensible amounts of healthier foods and smaller amounts of higher carb foods, higher fat, and higher calorie foods.

It's simple to do: draw an imaginary line down the middle of a dinner plate. Divide one half into two parts. Now there are 3 divisions on the plate.

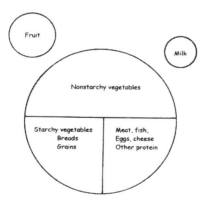

The biggest section should be filled with vegetables: that includes salad and cooked vegetables. Good choices would be:

asparagus	carrots	greens	radishes
beets	cauliflower	mushrooms	tomatoes
bok choy	celery	onions	turnips
broccoli	cucumber	pea pods	vegetable juice
cabbage	green beans	peppers	zucchini

One of the smaller areas is for a starchy vegetable such as a serving of:

cooked beans (pinto, kidney, etc.)	potatoes
bean soup	rice
corn	winter squash
peas	grits

The last area is for protein foods such as meat, fish, other seafood, or skinless poultry–the size of a deck of cards. Eggs, low fat cheese, or tofu would also be good choices in this section.

Next to the plate place a glass of milk (nonfat or 1%). For those who don't drink milk, they could add another small serving of a carbohydrate food such as a small roll, slice of bread, 1/2 pita, or light yogurt.

Lastly, also next to the plate, goes a serving of fruit (either a piece of fresh fruit or a dish with 1/2 cup unsweetened canned or frozen fruit).

At breakfast, half the plate is for starchy foods (bread, 1/2 cup cooked cereal, 3/4 cup most dry cereals, a 6-inch tortilla, or 1 4-in waffle or pancake).

Fruit in one small section could include: 1/2 banana, 1/2 cup juice, 1/2 cup fruit, an apple, peach, cup of melon or berries, etc.

The last section would have a protein food such as meat or a meat substitute (1 egg or egg substitute), 2 Tbsp. peanut butter, 1 oz. nuts, 1/2 cup tofu, or 1/4 cup cottage cheese.

The plate method works best with a 9-inch plate, instead of the usual 12-inch plate.

The goal is to increase fruits and vegetables and decrease animal-based foods which are usually higher in fat, especially saturated fat.

Portion Sizes

For people like Anthony who are newly diagnosed, on no medication and are overweight, rationing carbs and restricting calories are the main considerations. To make sure he doesn't eat too many calories, Anthony needs to learn what portion sizes are compatible with good blood sugar control and what kinds of foods have the most nutritional value with the least calories. Part of the dietitian's job is to teach Anthony what a sensible piece of meat looks like (one meat choice is one ounce, so the usual three-choice meat portion is only the size of a deck of cards). Most of us are not accustomed to thinking of that as a serving. Restaurants and butcher shops have trained us to expect BIG, THICK SLABS as normal. Bagels have "grown" from their former 2-choice size to 2-fisted "giants" of 4 to 5 carb choices. To educate Anthony, the dietitian showed him plastic models of food servings. She also urged him to measure his food with measuring cups (or on a small scale) at home for a while to learn what appropriate amounts look like.

Here are some visual cues of portion sizes that Anthony, or you, can take anywhere:

3 oz. meat = deck of cards
1 cup = fist or tennis ball
1 teaspoon butter, margarine, or peanut butter = tip of thumb
2 tablespoons = thumb
3 oz. fish = checkbook
2 Tbsp. mayo, oil, or dip = thumb
1 oz. cheese = 4 dice
medium potato = computer mouse
1 serving fruit = ½ tennis ball
1 serving pasta = ½ tennis ball
oatmeal = ice cream scoop
cold cereal = teacup to a fist

Timing

Often the dietitian works with the physician to balance meal times with the action times of insulin or diabetes pills. Even with Anthony, who is not on any diabetes medication, timing is of concern to the dietitian. That's where snacks can help.

The Role of Snacks

Snacks can serve several purposes.

1. They can keep blood sugar from going too low. Frequently, three meals a day are not sufficient to balance the peak action times of some insulins or pills. To prevent a low blood sugar due to medication, the dietitian may reserve some food servings from meals for one or two or three snacks. *These snacks are not treats to be*

added or left out on a whim. They prevent insulin or pills from lowering blood sugar too much between meals.

2. Snacks can keep blood sugar from going too high. I know that seems odd but it's true. Several hours after the last meal, the liver releases sugar to keep the blood sugar from going too low. If it didn't, we'd often faint between meals. For people with diabetes, the liver may release too much sugar when more than 4 to 5 hours go by between meals. By shortening the intervals between meals with snacks, we let the brain do the thinking about how much food (fuel) the body needs and keep the liver from doing it's own thing, sometimes badly.

3. Snacks can prevent overeating. For people who like to eat frequently, the dietitian might plan between-meal snacks to prevent hunger pangs that could lead a desperate "grazer" to go off the meal plan.

4. In Anthony's case a bedtime snack was written into his meal plan because of his personal preference.

Eating Meals on a Schedule

Even if someone takes pills or insulin, scheduling mealtimes can be *somewhat* flexible. While it's not possible to safely skip a meal when one is on some insulins or pills, a plan can usually be designed with a wide array of meal sizes and times. Everything from a small early breakfast, to a big late lunch to a light supper, to no snacks, to three snacks, or almost any combination you can think of, can usually be accommodated.

For people who work unusual hours, such as evening or night shifts, meals can be divided to adapt to this pattern, but long periods (more than 5 hours) without food (except during sleep) should be minimized. What *can't* be done easily for many people with diabetes is to change the agreed upon meal plan schedule by more than 30 minutes to an hour on a moment's notice.

Needing to eat on time is one of the main gripes people with diabetes have. And it's not just irksome for the person with diabetes. It causes countless problem situations with friends and family members, and sometimes colleagues and managers at work, who don't understand that eating on time is not just a personal quirk or a bid for control, but a medical necessity.

Sugar and Sugar-Free Foods

It's easy to assume that any food that says "sugar free" is okay for someone with diabetes. Wrong. Another common error is to think that "sugar-free" means there is no carbohydrate in the food. What "sugar-free" means, technically, (and this is how many food companies use the term on packages) is that the food has no granulated sugar (sucrose). But it may have corn syrup or fructose (fruit sugar), or any one of several other sugars (galactose, lactose, maltose, and glucose), or some other sweetener that has calories and can raise blood sugar to some degree.

Another labeling requirement is that the ingredient used in the largest amount be listed first, the next greatest is listed next, and so on. Sometimes food companies use several different sweeteners so no one sweetener is present in sufficient quantities to require having it at or near the top of the list of ingredients. Manufacturers hope this gives consumers the false impression that the product has negligible amounts of "sugary" sweeteners when the total amount might actually be quite significant.

More on Diet Foods

There's probably a section in your supermarket set aside for dietetic foods, which you might think would be a dandy place to find lots of food for people with diabetes.

The first problem with foods labeled "dietetic" is that "dietetic" does not mean "diabetic." A dietetic product may be for a low sodium, gluten free or some other diet and not be designed for a diabetic's needs at all. Also, even if some products are made with the person with diabetes in mind by using artificial sweeteners instead of some type of sugar, surprisingly, most of them are not low-calorie. A candy bar made for those with diabetes has just as much fat in it as a normal candy bar. Only the sugar is missing, and by now you know that most people with diabetes need to watch their fat and calories as much as their sugar intake.

Most dietetic products, except for sugar-free gelatin, sugar-free sodas, diet jelly and fat-free salad dressings are no great improvement over regular foods in moderation. Some dietetic foods cannot be used in significant quantities for two reasons: first, some of the artificial sweeteners such as sorbitol, can cause diarrhea, and, second, the saturated fat in chocolates and other dessert products can contribute to high cholesterol levels. Alas, a truly "harmless" diabetic dessert (except, perhaps, sugar-free gelatin) has not yet been invented.

Is It Sugar and Is It Bad?

Unlike coffee, tea, and diet sodas, which don't raise blood sugar, all foods such as starches and especially sugars do, to some degree. Table sugar, honey, corn syrup, maple syrup, etc. used to be thought of as invariably quick raisers of blood sugar and therefore to be avoided except to treat low blood sugar.

However, new nutrition research has shown that although these sweeteners may raise blood sugar quickly when eaten alone, if they are taken in small to moderate quantities with a meal containing fat, protein, and complex carbohydrates such as whole wheat pasta, they don't necessarily cause the blood sugar to rise sharply. The trick, though, is that they must be eaten in small amounts, eaten with a meal, and something else with carbohydrate may need to be omitted to accommodate the carbohydrates in the treat.

Although sugar may not be "bad" or forbidden, sugar and similar sweeteners provide little or no nutritional benefit and have significant calories. Health foods they aren't.

How Desserts Can Be Part of a Sensible Diabetic Meal

In the sample dinner Anthony wrote for his dietitian, he was entitled to have four carbohydrate choices, two of which he "met" with 1 cup of potatoes. Instead of the potatoes, though, he could have had a slice of angel food cake without frosting or 1/2 cup sherbet. Because these desserts are concentrated sources of carbohydrate, the portion sizes are, necessarily, small. Even if Anthony were willing to carefully limit himself to these small portions, it still wouldn't be a good idea for him to "trade away" potatoes every day to make room for a sweet dessert. The dessert has no significant nutritional value, whereas potatoes have complex carbohydrate, potassium, and fiber. Still, it's reasonable to eat desserts occasionally, and having the freedom to have treats makes for a greater willingness to stick to a meal plan.

This trading of one food for another may explain how your friend or family member with diabetes has claimed to be staying on their meal plan when you thought he or she was "cheating." The person may very well have been within the guidelines set by the dietitian.

The Glycemic Index

The system of categorizing foods according to how quickly and how far they raise blood sugar is called the Glycemic Index or GI. The GI shows that white and wheat bread raise the blood sugar higher in three hours than does ice cream. That's largely because the fat in the ice cream slows down its absorption. And regular potatoes raise it higher than sweet potatoes.

The GI is improved upon when the *quantity of carbohydrate* in the food is added to the GI calculation. That gives a more useful measure–the glucose load.

Most people with diabetes don't rely much on the GI to pick isolated foods because they rarely eat a food by itself. For example, they don't usually eat bread alone–they eat it as part of a sandwich or with a meal. Also, an individual's reaction to a carbohydrate is just that–individual. In a Tufts University study *GI responses to a particular food varied widely among individuals and differed significantly in the same people each of the three times they were tested.*

The American Diabetes Association position: "The use of the glycemic index and glycemic load may provide a modest additional benefit over that observed when total carbohydrate is considered alone."

People with diabetes, by testing their blood after eating, can learn from experience what foods raise their blood sugars and avoid them or eat them in small amounts with other foods.

What Form a Food Is In Matters

The greatest practical help of the research that resulted in the Glycemic Index is that we now know that the form the food is in makes a difference. It seems that the more pureed the food is, the quicker it is absorbed. Cooking also speeds up the transformation to sugar, as does eating a food on an empty stomach. In short, eating a raw chunk of food (like an apple) will raise blood sugar less than eating a cooked, pureed food (like applesauce) by itself. And apple juice raises blood sugar faster than either applesauce or a whole apple.

Salt

Salt is primarily made up of the minerals sodium and chloride and is the primary contributor of sodium in our diets. Most people use the terms interchangeably.

Since the body works best with a certain concentration of sodium, if there is too much, the kidneys try to dilute it by making less urine and retaining more water. More water in the blood vessels means more pressure against the sides of those vessels, causing increased blood pressure. Sometimes the body retains so much water that the ankles and even the whole body can swell. This swelling is called edema. High blood pressure and edema cause the heart to work harder to push that extra fluid around. Also, as you'll see in Chapter 11 on complications, high blood pressure is bad for the kidneys and bad for the eyes.

We'd get all the salt we needed from healthy foods if we never picked up a saltshaker the rest of our lives. Reducing salt is even more important, the older we get. As we age, the kidneys lose more and more of their ability to regulate sodium and fluid.

High blood pressure is almost always without symptoms so you'd only find out that it was high if it were checked. Because high blood pressure is often associated with fluid retention, it might mean that your kidneys were not regulating salt well.

A low salt diet is strongly recommended for someone with high blood pressure, congestive heart failure, cirrhosis of the liver, kidney disease, and for people taking certain medications like steroids.

The best advice is to cut down on salt. The recommended maximum amount of sodium is 1,500 to 2,400 mg per day. Unfortunately, the U.S. average intake is 3,500 to 4,000 mg. Anthony has slightly elevated blood pressure so his dietitian encouraged him to decrease his intake of sodium. But putting down the salt shaker will really provide only a small benefit. Most sodium in foods comes from processed foods such as canned and frozen foods, lunch meats, chips, crackers, cheese, salad dressings, soy sauce and restaurant foods. Anthony plans to buy more fresh vegetables, bake a chicken and use it in sandwiches instead of lunch meats, and cut down on eating out.

People who have given up salt on their doctor's orders usually say that in a few short weeks they find canned foods and other processed foods taste too salty. They don't miss the salt at all.

Reducing sodium can be relatively painless, so please think about making this positive change for yourself and your loved ones, with or without diabetes.

More Good News: Fiber

Fiber is a food ingredient that influences blood sugar–and a lot more. Its benefits include:

- Increasing the effectiveness of insulin;
- Delaying and smoothing the adsorption of sugars from the digestive tract;
- Lowering blood pressure;
- Promoting weight loss (by making you feel full longer after eating);
- Helping prevent colon, breast and ovarian cancers;
- Helping prevent constipation, diverticulosis and hemorrhoids.

Fiber is available only from plant foods. For example, there is no fiber in meat no matter how chewy it is.

There are two types of fiber, insoluble and soluble. Insoluble fiber is present in whole-wheat products, wheat and corn bran, and many vegetables. It's called insoluble because it holds on to water but it doesn't dissolve in it. These qualities help it move foods through the digestive tract faster, reducing exposure of the intestines' walls to cancer-causing agents in food. Its ability to attract water into the digestive tract also softens stools and helps prevent constipation.

Soluble fiber, the type found in dried beans and peas, oats, barley and many fruits and vegetables (such as apples, oranges and carrots) dissolves in water. It becomes like a gel and slows down the whole process of absorption through the wall of the intestine. Glucose is also more slowly absorbed in the presence of soluble fiber so the usual rise of the blood glucose level, especially right after meals, is more gradual. Thus, soluble fiber can help keep blood sugar levels more stable. Soluble fiber also decreases blood cholesterol and other blood fats.

Most North Americans don't eat enough fiber. We generally average only about 11 grams of fiber a day instead of 25-35 grams that many experts recommend. It's not hard to get enough fiber when we eat mostly vegetables, fruits and foods made from whole grains (all rich in one or both types of fiber). But since we don't, the easiest way to get a lot of fiber is to start the day with a bowl of high fiber cereal. Not all cereals are good sources of fiber. Cereals with double-digit amounts of fiber grams per serving are excellent sources–cereals with "high fiber" or "bran" in their names may not be. Comparing the fiber in one cereal with another can be hard. The cereal makers get to decide the portion size so they vary a lot from one cereal to the next. Sometimes you have to do some math. I've done some of the math for you so the following cereals are arranged in order from the most concentrated in fiber to those with very little.

Grams of Fiber in 100 Calories of Breakfast Cereal

All Bran Extra Fiber	26	Grape Nuts	3
Fiber One	24	Shredded Wheat	3
Kashi Go Lean	7	Frosted Mini Wheats	3
High Fiber O's	6	Wheaties	3
Raisin Bran	5	Oatmeal	3
Shredded Wheat n' Bran	4	Multi-Grain Cheerios	2
Oat Bran hot cereal	4	Fruit & Fiber	2
Total Whole Grain	3	Corn Flakes	1
Cheerios	3	Special K	1

Fiber is listed on food labels under "total carbohydrate" as "dietary fiber." Although, it's a part of carbohydrate, it's mostly indigestible and only some is absorbed. Currently, we teach our patients who are carb counting that if a food has 5 grams of fiber or more, they can subtract *half* of the grams of fiber from the total carbohydrate. Just a couple of years ago, we told people they could subtract *all* the fiber. But the latest research shows that only half the fiber isn't absorbed, the other half should be counted as part of the carbohydrate. Buyer beware, though, the diet food industry has chosen to stay with the old "subtract all the fiber" information. So you will still see some protein bars, and most foods claiming to be low carb, with a carbohydrate amount that may be suspiciously low.

Transitioning to Healthier Foods

One of the hardest tasks in getting used to healthier versions of familiar foods is the "taste shock." There are ways to make this easier.

My husband knew he should give up his beloved 2% milk and switch to 1% but he just didn't like it. What he finally did was pour 1 cup of milk out of the 2% carton of milk and replace it with 1% milk. He found that it tasted pretty much like it usually did. A couple of weeks later, he made a half and half mix (2 cups of each in the carton). Next he made a 1 cup 2% to 3 cups 1% mix. Finally, he was drinking all 1% milk and it was fine. The change was gradual enough.

The same technique could be used for pouring regular and sugar free sodas in a glass, or blending fat free with regular salad dressing.

If whole wheat bread is the problem, try a sandwich with one slice of your family member's old favorite and one slice with whole wheat. Who said both slices of a sandwich have to be made with the same bread?

Lastly, eating high fiber cereal is a great health habit. But there are two problems. First, nobody loves Fiber One or All Bran at first bite. Second, if someone switches from Shredded Wheat to All Bran from one day to the next, he will spend all day on the toilet and say really bad things about the person who talked him into switching. Maybe *you*. Fiber has to added gradually.

So sprinkle a couple tablespoonfuls of All Bran or Fiber One on that favorite cereal. Do that for a week. Add more the next week. Then start taking away some of the Shredded Wheat, or whatever, as you add more All Bran. Stop at any point. Even half and half is a great improvement over a low fiber cereal.

Food That's Good For People With Diabetes Is Good For Everybody

There are many more similarities than differences in what we should be eating and what someone with diabetes should be eating. Instead of setting people with diabetes apart as a deprived group that can't eat what we eat because they are "sick," we should be looking to them as models of how *to eat so as not to get sick.*

What Nutritionists Recommend For:

People *with* Diabetes	**People *without* Diabetes**
Low fat, especially low saturated fat	Low fat, especially low saturated fat
Zero trans fat	Zero trans fat
High fiber	High fiber
Moderate protein	Moderate protein
High complex carbohydrates	High complex carbohydrates
Low concentrated sugar	Low concentrated sugar
Low salt (possibly)	Low salt (possibly)
Calories to maintain a sensible weight	Calories to maintain a sensible weight

There is no difference in these two lists because eating low fat, high fiber, moderate protein, high carbohydrate (but not the ones with low nutritional value like sugar), possibly low salt and just enough calories to maintain a sensible weight, is the prescription for preventing numerous diseases. The number one cause of death in North America is still cardiovascular disease. Nursing homes are full of people disabled by strokes. High cholesterol and high levels of fat in the blood, plus high blood pressure exacerbated by high salt diets are implicated in heart disease and strokes. Colon cancer is more prevalent in people who eat high fat, low fiber diets. But it doesn't have to happen, at least not at the relatively young ages that heart attacks and strokes and cancer are felling us.

The sensible person with diabetes and all health-conscious non-diabetics should be eating the same foods. So find a person with diabetes who is taking good care of himself and eat what he eats!

7

Inviting Someone With Diabetes
To Your Home For A Meal

Have you ever invited someone with diabetes to your home for a meal and then felt uncertainty and panic, wondering what to serve? My neighbor Beth came to me with that problem. Her brother was bringing his girlfriend, Patty, over for the Fourth of July family barbecue and Beth was panicky about what to serve.

Beth doesn't need to wriggle out of hosting the party, or prepare two menus, or buy everything in the dietetic section of her supermarket.

In this chapter we will discuss what questions to ask your guest with diabetes before meal plans are finalized. There are samples of good and not-so-good menus, examples of ways to reduce sugar and fat and suggestions on where to find recipes and other specific helps round out this guide.

To get back to helping Beth, she will feel a lot more confident if she calls Patty to find out *what* Patty can eat and *when* she needs to eat. In fact, that's the first thing you should do if you want to avoid misunderstandings.

Ask If Timing Is Important

The first question to ask is, "Do you need to eat at a certain time?" Once you have agreed on a time for dinner, ask, "Is it important that we stay with that exact time or do you have some leeway?" Time is usually important for someone taking oral medication to lower blood sugar and some types of insulins. Briefly this is because these medications are taken in advance with the expectation that food will be eaten to coincide with their peak action times. Without food at those peaks, blood sugar can get too low.

People who control their diabetes solely by diet and exercise have fewer constraints placed on their eating schedule. At the other end of the treatment spectrum are those who inject insulin with every meal and those who wear an insulin pump that gives insulin whenever it's needed. They don't have to match their food to their insulin schedule because they're matching their insulin to their food schedule. They take insulin shortly before the food will be served, so if they know about a delay ahead of time, they can hold off on taking their insulin.

Patty's answer to Beth about this question was that it would be easiest for her to eat between 5:00 and 6:00 since this was her usual evening meal hour. She added that she could make some adjustments if that wasn't convenient.

Beth was glad she'd asked since it was no problem to schedule the dinner for around 5:30. She was especially glad because Patty sounded very pleasantly surprised that Beth had bothered to call, and Patty's "thanks for asking" was nice to hear.

Ask About Food Restrictions

In this day of allergies and diets for all kinds of medical conditions, from allergies to ulcers, it is a kindness to ask any guest if they have any special food needs you should consider in planning the meal.

If you asked a hundred people with diabetes what they could and couldn't eat, you would likely get fifty different answers. You could hear anything from, "Don't fuss, I can eat the same food you can," to "I can eat anything low-fat that doesn't have sugar in it."

A person with diabetes might not be willing to eat:
Desserts made with sugar
Foods made with honey, corn syrup, or barbecue sauce
Regular maple syrup, jams and jellies
Foods high in protein (meat, fish and dairy products)
Foods high in fat (butter, margarine, fatty meats, mayonnaise, cheese, cream, salad dressing, etc.)

A person with diabetes *may* be willing to eat:
Desserts made with artificial sweeteners (Splenda, Equal, and SugarTwin)

Desserts made with sugar (in small quantities)
Vegetables cooked with little or no sugar or fat
Salads with low-fat dressing
Syrups and jams made with artificial sweeteners (just because it says "Lite" or "no added sugar" is *not* automatically okay–ask or read the label carefully and compare it with regular products to see if there's really a difference.)
Bread
Foods that are boiled, steamed or baked without added fat
Pasta, rice and potatoes without fatty sauces and toppings
Lean meat, poultry and fish

Again, the varieties of responses you may get are a result of different treatment plans and different goals. Treatment can change over time, too, so you'll want to get current information. For example, the relative you invite today may need to be very rigid about food choices because of the need to maintain a certain blood sugar or protect his kidneys or keep his blood pressure down. However, a few months ago, he may not have had the same motivation or the same medical necessity.

Imagine your friend or relative with diabetes at a get-together where the only thing served that he or she can eat is tossed salad or veggies with no dressing, and the only thing to drink without sugar or alcohol is water.

This could happen if the menu was one of these:

Menu #1: A Barbecue
Chips and onion dip
Barbecued ribs
Potato Salad
Coleslaw
Macaroni salad
Cornbread
Tossed salad
Ranch dressing
Ice cream sundaes
Regular soda
Wine and beer

Menu #2: Dinner for Company
Cream of mushroom soup
Prime rib roast
Creamed onions
Twice-baked potatoes
Buttered broccoli
Raw vegetable plate
Hot rolls
Apple pie
Wine
Coffee

In Menu #1, the person who is watching fat and cholesterol intake is left with the tossed salad, and that may have to be with little or no dressing unless the host provides a low-fat salad dressing. All the other salads are high in fat from mayonnaise or sour cream, and the cornbread contains considerable fat and sugar. The chips, dip, and ribs are all fatty so they are not a good idea (except for tiny tastes). There is no available sugar-free soda, so the only safe beverages are one glass of wine or beer (if the calories and alcohol in the wine or beer are not a problem) and water. Plain coffee and tea do not have calories or raise blood sugar. However, coffee creamers are high in sugar and fat and flavored gourmet coffee blends may be also.

Menu #2 contains lots of fat and a dessert high in both fat and sugar. For careful people, only the raw vegetables and a hot roll or two plus coffee can be eaten in normal quantities without guilt or problems. Everything else has to be taken in very small portions or skipped.

Here are some of the comments I hear from people with diabetes about choices when eating with friends and family.

"It would be thoughtful if they would have things
I can have as well, such as diet soda."

"Tell me if it is made with sugar or other sweeteners and, if so, how much. I don't like surprises.

"I wish people knew how much I appreciated them offering alternative desserts.

What Should You Serve?

What's the answer? I recommended to my neighbor Beth that she start with a heart-healthy menu that would be good for everyone, including herself. (Alternatively, she could keep the fatty foods and add a couple of extra items to the menu that are low in fat and sugar).

For example, at the barbecue where Menu #1 is to be served, Beth could have skinless chicken breast or low-fat hot dogs like Oscar Mayer Light Beef Franks or Morningstar Farms Grillers Original veggie burgers (See Recipes in the Appendix). She could have plain bread or rolls (most have little or no fat). For dessert she could serve a fruit salad with whipped topping or ice cream on the side. Offering a selection of salad dressings, including a low-fat or nonfat variety, is a considerate touch. At my urging, Beth also decided to have sugar-free soda, including one with no caffeine, since this is also an ingredient many people try to avoid, for reasons unrelated to diabetes.

Although Patty would have enough choices with the preceding changes, I proposed that Beth try to serve a meal that would be healthier for everyone–for Patty, for Beth's parents and in-laws who are in their 60's, for Beth and her sister and brother who have been battling their weight for years, for her husband with the borderline high cholesterol, and for her kids.

This is the menu that Beth created and which I heartily approved:

A Better Barbecue Menu
Raw vegetable platter with low-fat dip
Marinated chicken breast kabobs
Grilled Idaho or sweet potatoes
Sliced tomatoes and cucumbers
Unsweetened fresh fruit salad
Whipped topping (on the side)
Sugar-free lemonade or diet soda
Regular soda
Wine and beer

Alternatives to Menu #2 include roast turkey or baked or broiled fish instead of the prime rib, baked potatoes with sour cream and butter on the side, unbuttered vegetables and a low-fat, low-sugar dessert such as a chiffon pie made with artificial sweetener (the *very* careful can eat only the filling and leave the crust) or a commercial low fat, sugar-free dessert like Dreyer's Slow-Churned No Sugar Added Ice Cream.

A Better Dinner For Company Menu
Minestrone soup
Broiled salmon with lemon slices
Hungarian green beans (recipe in Appendix)
Baked potatoes with topping on the side
Mixed green salad
Regular and low-fat dressings on the side
Dinner roll
Butter
Mixed berry cup with low fat ice cream on the side
Sugar-free soda or mineral water with lemon slice
Wine
Coffee and tea

Beverages

Sugar-free sodas are very popular and will be welcome to most people with diabetes. Beware when shopping, however. There are some flavored sparkling waters and clear sodas that look as though they are sugar free but aren't. They are sweetened with high-fructose corn syrup. Many have almost as much sugar and calories as regular soda pop. *Check the label carefully* for ingredients and look for a drink that is *unsweetened* or *artificially* sweetened.

Alcohol is another tricky beverage. It can lead to severely low blood sugars if drunk without a meal or if drunk to excess even with food. (For more about the low blood sugar dangers of alcohol see Chapter 8 on dining out).

In addition to the safety issue, alcohol has a surprisingly high number of calories, almost as many as fat. One and a half ounces of hard liquor, 4 ounces of wine, or 12 ounces of beer each have the equivalent of two fat choices or about 90 calories from the alcohol portion alone. Wine and beer have still more calories from the carbohydrate they also contain.

Yet another disadvantage of alcohol is that it can make people forget their diets and pile on the wrong foods.

A considerate host or hostess may offer, but should never push alcohol.

Dessert

Don't automatically include a recipe or a commercial product because of broad terms like "diabetic dessert." Many recipes and diabetic foods are geared toward the younger, insulin-dependent person with diabetes who may not have a weight problem and who may only be concerned about limiting sugars and other carbohydrates.

Most diabetic desserts have almost as many calories as ordinary sweets. In most cases, all the fat has been left in the candies, cookies, and cake mixes, and it's the fat that primarily raises the calorie count.

Since 3/4s of the people with diabetes need to watch their calorie and fat intake as much as their sugar, high-fat commercial foods and recipes that call for a 1/2 cup or more of butter or cream cheese are not acceptable even if they are artificially sweetened.

This again emphasizes the importance of asking what your guest's restrictions are and not making assumptions.

Sugar: It Can Be Sneaky

Chances are good, though, that you'll be asked to use little or no sugar at least in part of the menu. That's trickier than you might imagine, since lots of substances are chemically sugars but are not known by that name.

Any sweetener that has calories can raise blood sugar. These caloric sweeteners have 4 calories a gram. That doesn't sound like much, but for ordinary granulated sugar, that translates into 770 calories per cup.

Some Other Names For Sugar

Molasses	Raw sugar	Corn syrup
Turbinado	Brown sugar	Starch syrup
Rice syrup	Tapioca syrup	Treacle
Honey	Refiners' syrup	Potato syrup
Glucose	Agave syrup	Maltose
Carob powder	Dextrose	Barley syrup
Dextrin	Sorghum syrup	High fructose corn syrup

Some people claim that because some of these sugars (e.g. honey) are not refined, they provide valuable nutrients. However, the amount of any nutrients in honey is so minuscule as to hardly matter.

Sugar alcohols are another group of sweeteners that have calories. They include: sorbitol, mannitol, dulcitol, and xylitol and are common in candies and gum labeled "sugar free." They are absorbed more slowly into the blood than sugar and therefore may cause a less dramatic blood sugar rise, especially in someone who is not completely dependent on injections for insulin. However, they can cause bloating and diarrhea when eaten in surprisingly small quantities. (The amount in a package of Tic Tacs or two sugar-free hard candies can cause discomfort.)

Lactose is a sugar put in milk by the cow. It is a natural and caloric sweetener. This milk sugar is why sugar is listed in the "Nutrition Facts" label on every dairy product in the section titled, "Total Carbohydrate."

Fructose is a natural sugar commonly found in fruits. It doesn't raise the blood sugar rapidly in well-controlled diabetes, but it has calories and must be counted as a carbohydrate. Note that while it doesn't raise blood sugar as rapidly, it does raise it, especially in people whose blood sugar is generally too high. Fructose is found in many dietetic products and commercial baked goods. There is no significant advantage to using fructose or the fruit juices commonly called for in older diabetic cookbooks. Your body can't really tell the difference between the sugar from an apple (or other fruit) and the sugar from a beet or cane.

Fructose has another problem. Studies have shown that fructose, along with table sugar, can contribute to higher LDL cholesterol (the bad kind) and triglyceride levels. Since people with diabetes are already more prone to high cholesterol and triglycerides and because the higher these blood fats are, the greater the risk of having a heart attack or stroke, anything that contributes to raising these should be used in moderation.

Syrups and other forms of glucose are common sweeteners in baked goods and commercial products. The syrup you've probably heard of most is corn syrup.

Food labels list ingredients in decreasing order of their quantity in the product. Try to steer clear of foods that have one of the above sugars or syrups as the first ingredient. Also avoid those that list several caloric sweeteners, no matter where they are on the list of ingredients. Even small amounts add up—some manufacturers use several different sweeteners to make it seem as though the total amount of sweeteners is less than it really is. They do this by using small enough quantities of each so that they appear lower in the list of ingredients.

Artificial Sweeteners

Some sweeteners that have no calories and that do not raise blood sugar are:

Sucralose (Splenda)
Equal (aspartame or NutraSweet)
Sweet One (acesulfame potassium or acesulfame-K)
Saccharin (SugarTwin, Sweet'N Low, etc.)
Stevia (Truvia, PureVia)
Cyclamates (not available in the U.S.)

Artificial Sweeteners Have Limitations

You can substitute non-caloric or artificial sweeteners for sugar, honey, and syrups in some recipes. Equal, however, loses its sweetness with prolonged heating, so it cannot be used in a baked cake, baked pie, or baked beans. It is able to withstand the heat of boiling water added to gelatin, though, or it can be added *after* a dish is cooked. It does not add the texture that is needed in some baked goods, which sugar provides in addition to sweetness.

For baking you can try SugarTwin, which has a bulking agent added for texture and saccharin for sweetness. The good news is that saccharin can be used in baking. The bad news is SugarTwin and other saccharine products can leave a bitter aftertaste.

Splenda can be used in baking. It comes in a granulated version with a bulking agent that measures cup for cup like sugar and also in a mixture that's half sugar. The half sugar mix gives the best results in texture and browning for baking, but the sugar adds significant calories and carbohydrate. Most people tell me Splenda has the least artificial sweetener aftertaste.

Artificial sweeteners substituted for sugar can enable a beverage or gelatin dessert to be carbohydrate and calorie free. Baked goods are not so "fortunate." For example, a typical blueberry muffin has four sources of carbohydrate: flour, sugar, blueberries and milk.

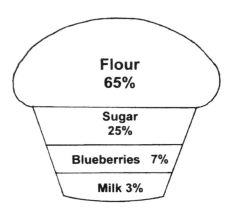

Flour
65%

Sugar
25%

Blueberries 7%

Milk 3%

As you can see, even if you substituted an artificial sweetener for all the sugar, and didn't mind that the muffin would likely be dry and gummy, you'd only reduce the carbohydrate by 25%. The flour is a much more significant source of carbohydrate. But until someone invents artificial flour, baked goods will continue to be large sources of carbohydrate even when made with an artificial sweetener.

Sugar In Moderation

Sugar does not have to be completely avoided. For many years, it was believed that simple sugar, like honey or table sugar, is responsible for quicker and higher rises in blood sugar than complex carbohydrates (starches) such as rice and potatoes. Recent research, however, suggests that the difference is not very significant.

So it is the total amount of carbohydrate (all the sugars and all the starches) that should be considered *in a meal*. Whether the person with diabetes gets the carbohydrate from bread, beans or maple syrup will not significantly change the high point of his or her blood sugar after the meal.

In theory this means that a diabetic could eat a dessert made with some granulated sugar instead of some or all of the bread, potatoes, pasta, milk, fruit, or any other food that contains carbohydrate. Notice the word "instead." No one with diabetes should eat the usual amount of carbohydrate at mealtime *and* add a sugary dessert. The result would be high blood sugar.

This fairly new idea is being greeted with mixed feelings. Some diabetics say they are quite sensitive to simple sugar and feel that they are better off without it.

Others welcome the greater freedom that "trading" can mean to them. It means they can eat a slice of birthday cake or a candy bar if they omit an equivalent amount of some other carbohydrate and maybe fat too.

The disadvantage of eating a candy bar or cake instead of a more nutritious food is that they would be trading empty sugar calories (and probably lots of saturated fat) for a serving of fiber, vitamins, minerals and other nutrients.

Another problem is that sugar is not called a concentrated sweet for nothing. It doesn't take much sugar to add up to a lot of a less concentrated carbohydrate.

For example, here's what a diabetic would have to trade away to eat just one tablespoon of sugar:

1 dinner roll (or)
1 slice of bread (or)
1 glass of milk (or)
3 cups popcorn

Each of these foods is a lot of nutritious food to give up for a food with one tablespoon of sugar. And if you consider that a single slice of chocolate cake with chocolate frosting has about 3¾ tablespoons of sugar, that 's equal to 11¼ cups of popcorn or, more realistically 3 cups of popcorn, 1 slice of bread, 1 glass of milk *and* a dinner roll!

Knowing the amount of sugar per serving would be a help to your guest in deciding what and how much to choose from several carbohydrates to equal his or her total carbohydrate ration. You can help your guest with diabetes keep a normal blood sugar and still enjoy the food you serve.

The easiest way to know the amount of carbohydrate in a dish is to use recipes that include this information. See Resources for some good cookbooks.

How To Reduce Fats In Foods

The most common sources of fat in food are dairy products, meats, and oils used in frying and dressings.

Milk and milk products can be high or low in fat. Here are some dairy products that have little or no fat:

Nonfat (skim) milk	Fat-free buttermilk
Nonfat dry milk	Nonfat yogurt
Nonfat sour cream	Evaporated skim milk
Nonfat or low fat (1%) cottage cheese	1% low fat milk

You may have wondered why cheese is not on the list. That's because regular cheese is so high in fat that it is considered more like a meat. In diabetes nutrition guides meats and cheeses are divided into high-fat, medium-fat, and lean meat groups depending on their fat content.

Most meats fall into the medium-fat category. Prime cuts of beef and almost all cheeses, such as American, Blue, Cheddar, Monterey and Swiss are in the high-fat group.

Your best choices will come from the lean meat substitutes listed here:

Canadian Bacon	Oysters
Chipped beef	Parmesan cheese
Chicken	Rabbit
Cornish hen	Shellfish
Fat-free or low fat cheese	Soy protein foods
Fish	Tenderloin
Flank steak	Tuna (fresh or canned in water)
Ham (fresh or boiled)	Turkey
Lunch meat (85% fat free)	Venison

Egg yolks have enough fat in them to put whole eggs into the medium-fat meat group. Yolks are also high in cholesterol so they should only be eaten, at most, three times a week. There are some healthy ways to use egg whites, however. Here are some low-fat options:

Egg Choices

Egg substitutes with less than 55 calories per ¼ cup can be used in baking, omelets, etc. (some egg substitutes are made of only egg whites and coloring, whereas others have added vegetable oil.

You'll need to read the label on the carton for the fat and calorie content).

Scrambled eggs or French toast can be made with 2 whites and 1 yolk.

The occasional whole egg should be poached, boiled or "fried" in a non-stick pan with Pam or other cooking spray.

Meat Portions

In addition to choosing a lean meat or lean meat substitute, you need to know how much is an allowable portion for a diabetic. You'll probably consider diabetic portions very small compared to what you're used to. Again, the usual diabetic meat portion is 3 ounces, which is about the size of a pack of playing cards. Some examples of 3-ounce meat portions are:

> ½ chicken breast
> 1 unbreaded fish fillet
> ¾ cup canned tuna in water
> 5 medium canned sardines
> 1 small hamburger patty

Meat Preparation Suggestions

1. To cook meat, don't fry–instead bake, boil, roast, or grill.
2. Trim off visible fat before and after cooking.
3. Do not add flour, breadcrumbs or coating mixes (they absorb fat).
4. Use a nonstick pan and nonstick spray to brown or "fry."
5. Cook meat or poultry on a rack so the fat will drain off.
6. Serve gravy or sauce on the side.

Miscellaneous Sources Of Fat

Other sources of fat besides meat, eggs, cheese and milk products are foods rich in vegetable fats. These include:

Avocado	Nondairy coffee creamer	Olives
Coconut	Peanut butter	Seeds (sunflower
Margarine	Vegetable shortening	pumpkin and pine
Nuts	Vegetable oil	nuts)

None of the above foods has cholesterol because all of them are plant products and cholesterol comes only from animals. But they are all high fat and some are 100% fat, so they are easily transformed into excess body fat. By limiting them as much as possible in the food you serve–you will be kind to yourself as well.

In addition to trying low-fat cooking techniques and new recipes, be on the lookout for new products in your market. The food industry regularly launches new fat-free and low-fat foods that make healthy eating increasingly sacrifice-free.

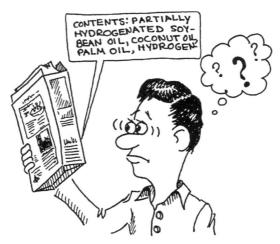

IT'S IMPORTANT TO READ LABELS
TO KNOW WHAT YOU'RE SERVING.

Consider Serving Size

What is healthy and what is not, is not only determined by the ingredient list. When you shop, look at the number of servings and the size of serving the product has. If you just look at the number of calories per serving, you could be fooled. Even potato chips don't seem bad at 145 calories per ounce. Most of us can afford a 145-calorie splurge a day. But if you notice that bag contains 12 ounces and the manufacturer says a serving is 1 ounce, you know that 145 calories is 1/12 the package! I don't know about you, but for many folks a normal serving size of potato chips would be ½ bag or 6 servings. Multiplying 145 by 6 equals 870 calories. So I don't buy or serve potato chips. Serving sizes printed on packages are notoriously skimpy. You need to estimate what *you* consider a realistic serving and calculate whether or not it is still a fat/calorie/sugar bargain.

What Should You Say If The Person With Diabetes Takes a "Bad" Food?

One of the most common complaints I hear from people with diabetes is that non-medical people without diabetes try to point out what they shouldn't be eating. Often the advice givers are wrong, especially if they are operating from the mistaken idea that no one with diabetes should ever eat sugar.

As has been mentioned, *small to moderate amounts* of sugar or honey or other blood sugar raising sweeteners actually may not be bad, provided they are eaten with a balanced meal and are calculated within the allowances for carbohydrate, protein, and fat for that meal.

So, raised eyebrows, shocked looks, shaking heads, and even a whispered, "Should you be eating that?" are generally infuriating to people with diabetes. When I asked what they do when someone tells them what to eat, they said:

> "It depends who is telling me. If it is family, I feel it is a direct challenge to me, so I many times want to do the opposite." (Laura, 43)

> "I do the opposite. I don't like others (parents, friends, etc.) controlling my diabetes. I have to live with it, they don't. They don't know what a diabetic goes through."
> (Samantha, 14)

> "It depends on who is talking. If it is my doctor, she knows what she is talking about. If it's a friend or someone else's parent, I ignore them." (Megan, 13)

"Usually those who comment know very little about the disease and are overweight and should be on a diet and watch what they eat themselves." (Anonymous)

"I don't want reminders." (Joan, 29)

"When my husband criticizes a poor eating choice (pie or cream, for instance), I bristle. But I know his criticism is warranted so although the immediate effect is resentment, the delayed effect is that it reinforces my resolve to avoid such foods as regular parts of my diet." (Elsa, 56)

Maybe your observation will have the long-term, positive effect that Elsa's husband's criticism has with her. But, judging from the responses I've gotten, it's more likely that you will irritate someone into doing just the opposite of what you're advising.

In short, what people with diabetes have asked me to tell you is that they will take care of it themselves. They will fill their plates or not, they will eat everything they've taken, or not, and they will eat cake or not. Until you have their level of knowledge about diabetes in general and their diabetes in particular, you should not be making any but the most diplomatic suggestions and probably not even those.

You want to help, though, so if you can't say things like, "Should you be eating that?" what can you do that they won't take wrong? Read on.

How To Help

In the area of food, the biggest help you can be to someone who has diabetes is to not sabotage their meal plan. I'm sure that would not be your intent, but it happens.

Mrs. Clark was an elderly widow from the South. She belonged to a church my diabetic friend Bob joined. Mrs. Clark loved to bake but she didn't get a chance to do it much after her husband died. He used to praise her pecan pies to the skies and she missed that, so she baked for every church event she could. She would hover over her pies and urge people to eat, and then urge them to eat some more. Of course they complimented her on her pecan pie (deservedly), while she beamed.

It wasn't enough to get ten or fifteen people to eat her pies, though. She wanted my friend Bob to "eat up" too. When he tried refusing, she looked sad. He tried taking only a taste, but when he wouldn't eat a whole piece she thought he didn't like her pie and was crushed. It didn't make any difference when he said he had diabetes. Her rejoinder was, "Oh, but it's only this once." Since Bob knew that a 430-calorie piece of pecan pie with 24 grams of fat and 52 grams of carbohydrate (which is more than he usually gets in his whole lunch) would send his blood sugar soaring, he stood firm.

Because he didn't do the easy thing and eat the pie to please Mrs. Clark, he was able to be tolerant of her efforts. But consider what his opinion of her, and himself as well, would have been if he had eaten the slice of pecan pie and found his blood sugar double his normal level when he checked it later.

Bob is likely to meet Mrs. Clark or someone like her again. One tack he, and you, can take is to find something else to praise besides their cooking. Your voice, added to his, can make a difference. And I wouldn't give up trying to educate the Mrs. Clarks about diabetes –she might decide to try her hand at low-fat, sugar-free desserts as a new challenge.

Instead of risking being a Mrs. Clark by having only pie or some other unhealthy old standby at your dinner, how about having fresh fruit available or a low-fat, artificially sweetened dessert that your family member or friend can have without guilt and without blood sugar elevations?

To find recipes for healthy dishes look in the Recipes section at the back of this book. Also try your library or bookstore for recently published cookbooks, the newer the better. Many books written in the last 10 years will give calorie and other nutritional information *plus* use available ingredients, including some new and improved products. Or ask your diabetic friends if they have a favorite dish they have been yearning for. You won't go wrong with *their* recipe.

When you serve your special recipe, though, don't make an issue of the fact that you went out of your way to produce this healthy dessert especially for your diabetic cousin Joan. First, you won't be alerting people that it's good for them, which might make them expect it to taste bad, but more importantly, Joan won't be embarrassed by having her different needs advertised. You and Joan need be the only ones who know what a saint you are. Being singled out for special attention (and notoriety) is not welcomed.

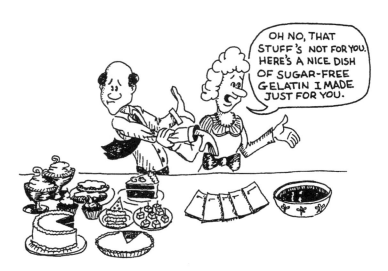

My friend Lisa was mortified at a dinner party when the hostess brought her her very own plate of food especially prepared according to a diabetes cookbook. Imagine the work that involved! Sadly, it was not appreciated. Lisa would have preferred to have what everybody else had. If something was not on her meal plan, she could have had a tiny taste and left the rest.

If I seem to be contradicting myself, let me clarify what people with diabetes want. Either make everything low fat, low-sugar, and so forth, or be ready to point out what the ingredients are *to everyone in ringing tones, or* to the person with diabetes in a discrete way.

At my last buffet dinner party, I had little notes stuck onto serving dishes that said things like "fat-free bean dip" and "sugar-free" on the whipped topping and the pumpkin pie. It did the job but didn't look very elegant. A guest who is famous for her entertaining skills suggested that I use place cards in decorative holders to identify the ingredients.

I know from experience that serving healthier foods can be more work. It is more time-consuming to choose, wash, cut up, and display a tray of veggies than to dump out a bag of chips and open a container of fatty sour cream dip. Anyone can take the easy way that is bad for people. After all, many of us have a file box full of recipes we shouldn't be using. Compiling a collection of healthy recipes that taste good is the challenge of today's cook. You can be different and be asked for your healthier recipes.

8

Dining Out With Someone With Diabetes

Lloyd, who has type 2 diabetes, told me about getting an invitation to go out after work. Since he was new in the office, he was pleased to be included in the group. But their plans caused him some concern. This is how the conversation went:

SUSAN: Lloyd, a bunch of us from accounting and personnel are planning to go out to dinner after work. Would you like to join us?

LLOYD: I sure would, what time will we eat and where?

SUSAN: Oh, we always go to the Big Drinks Lounge for three-dollar drinks at happy hour. We decide later where and when to eat dinner–that is, if we don't feel full after pretzels and peanuts. If we go to a restaurant afterwards, it's usually to Gus's Grease Garden or the Stupendous Steak.

Why is Lloyd concerned about these plans? What's wrong with cocktails before dinner, a to-be-decided-later-dinner time, and the restaurant choices? In this chapter we will also discuss why even a little alcohol without a meal can be dangerous for someone with diabetes, how easy it is to confuse a low blood sugar with over-indulgence in alcohol, and why mealtimes need to be on schedule. We'll discuss the right questions to ask a diabetic and how to help others who don't have diabetes understand why keeping to a timetable for meals is not just a whim. By supporting the person with diabetes you will lessen the likelihood that he or she will fail to ask the server about ingredients and cooking methods and keep mum about an unhealthy restaurant choice. For example, he might be tempted to jettison his meal plan to "be one of the gang."

Choosing the right restaurant and making the right menu selections can help the person with diabetes stay on a healthy diet.

As we discussed in Chapter 6, what a diabetic eats is an important part of his or her treatment plan. In general, eating healthily means reducing fat, calories, sodium, and sugar, and increasing vegetables, grains, and fresh fruits.

You Too Can Eat Wisely

I do hope that you too, are making some of these healthier choices for yourself, at least when you are with this special person. Even if you don't have an immediate medical reason to restrict your fat or salt or sugar, doing so will benefit you in the long run. You will also be setting a good example, will make your friend or family member with diabetes feel less different, and you'll save them from casting yearning looks at what is on your plate and feeling deprived.

Alcohol And Diabetes

You might spare Lloyd some discomfort if you can help avoid the happy hour scene. The free hors d'oeuvres are almost always unhealthy and the drinks are not a good idea for Lloyd either.

When a person with diabetes drinks alcohol his or her blood sugar can become too low, with serious consequences.

Low blood sugar is not only uncomfortable, it can cause falls and auto accidents, even without alcohol. Just as critical, however, is the potential for mistaking the symptoms of low blood sugar for being "under the influence." Symptoms of low blood sugar include poor coordination and slurred speech. Add another symptom, confusion, and you have someone who looks and acts like they're drunk. When any of us drink alcohol, our liver concentrates on processing the alcohol and stops providing us with the between-meal sugar that helps keep the blood sugar level from getting too low.

It is possible for a diabetic to drink a glass of wine with dinner because the food will keep the blood sugar from getting too low, so the reserve supply in the liver will not be needed. One or, at most, two drinks can be safely consumed–but only with a meal.

Even if the diabetic eats while he or she is drinking, there is a limit to how long the food will maintain the blood sugar level when more than one or two drinks are consumed. What happens when the food stops working, and the liver is still "off duty" working on the alcohol? What if the result is a very low blood sugar at 3 a.m. with no one around to observe it and do what's necessary? His or her sleep could become permanent.

Moderation is essential, and for someone with diabetes, moderation means one or two drinks. There is no safe way for a person with diabetes to drink more.

A final point about alcoholic drinks is to remember that they're fattening–almost as fattening as pats of butter. Most people with type 2 diabetes are trying to lose weight, and the addition of drinks to a meal means excess calories. Hopefully, the person trying to lose weight will choose a diet soda or water instead of wine, beer or whiskey. Twisting the person's arm to join you in an alcoholic beverage is another push towards loss of control.

Scheduling A Time

Meal *time* is just as important when eating out as when you invite someone to your home to eat. Again, ask the person with diabetes, "Once we agree on a time for dinner, is it important that we stay with that time?

Scheduling includes knowing if the restaurant you're considering is still in business, checking the hours it's open, making reservations, if appropriate, and knowing the traffic will let you get there within an hour of the diabetic's expected dinnertime.

If your car breaks down or there is an extreme road condition that gets you stuck in traffic, Lloyd will manage with the snacks he usually carries, or he'll tell you if you need to get him some juice, soda or food. My point is that everyone will be happier if the *preventable* inconveniences are avoided.

Choosing The Restaurant

Dining out means no one in the party has to do the cooking but *it doesn't relieve the planner from considering the kind of restaurant.* Any restaurant will have healthy and unhealthy menu choices. But certain types of restaurants will have more options for a health-conscious person with or without diabetes.

Chinese

Although Chinese restaurants have some less healthy items, such as fried egg rolls, fried wontons, butterfly shrimp, and sweet and sour pork, most dishes use the stir-fry method with little or no sugar and very little oil. You can even request that the "dry wok" cooking method be used. Numerous entrees are mainly vegetables, with only a little meat added for flavor. Chinese restaurants have many healthy options but you or someone with diabetes still must ask what is deep-fried and what has sugar, at least until you have settled on some safe favorite dishes.

The downside is the sodium level. A mere tablespoon of soy sauce, a basic ingredient in many Chinese dishes, has over 1,000 mg of sodium (about half a day's recommended maximum). Even a low-sodium version has about 600 mg per tablespoon.

Thai, Vietnamese, Indian and Japanese

Some good Asian cuisines, in addition to Chinese, are Indian, Thai, Vietnamese, and Japanese (skip the deep-fried tempura and opt for the sukiyaki, sushi and vegetables). Most Thai dishes are stir-fried, steamed, boiled or barbecued, but try to avoid duck, cashews, peanut sauce, coconut milk–all extremely fatty–and the highly sugared iced tea.

Mexican

Although Mexican restaurants start out with some healthy ingredients like beans and salsa, they are famous for their deep-fried foods, cheese toppings, sour cream, avocado and lard-laden tortillas. It's tough to eat healthily at a Mexican restaurant. It *can* be done by being very picky and creative, for example, by ordering a taco salad with no meat or avocado but lots of salsa. Have the cheese and sour cream served on the side, and leave most of the cheese and sour cream, along with the fried shell, on the plate. And skip the nacho chips! See what I mean about being picky? Mexican restaurants make healthy ordering significantly more difficult.

Fast Food

It used to be that fast-food restaurants had nothing for people who were trying to eat healthily. But even McDonald's now has main meal salads with grilled chicken. Almost every other fast food restaurant has some kind of *grilled (ask to be sure it's not fried)* chicken sandwich. To be really on track, if calories are an issue, you still have to scrape off some of the mayo and beware of fried anything. One of the best additions to most menus is a side salad with low-fat dressing–an excellent substitute for fries.

Ordering, for anyone concerned about fat, calories, sodium or carbohydrates, has been made easier by the online and printed nutrition summaries most fast-food places now offer. You may have to ask for a copy because they are not always displayed.

Coffee Shop Breakfast

Almost no combination or special on a breakfast menu is low in fat. Even if bacon, fried eggs, omelets, sausage, waffles and French toast are skipped, it's hard to order healthily. Croissants have buttery dough, muffins have lots of oil, and hash browns are just another name for fried potatoes.

Breakfast is best ordered from the side order section. There you and your friend can get oatmeal or cold cereal with nonfat milk, a fruit cup and toast (butter on the side).

Alternatively, pancakes ordered without butter are relatively low in fat and most restaurants have sugar-free maple syrup for your friend with diabetes. There's nothing that says *you* can't have *your* pancakes with it too. You probably won't like it as well as regular syrup, but your willingness to try it and your ease at letting the waitress think *you're* different are good demonstrations of the fact that you two are a team. It also shows your friend or family member with diabetes what is available and how to get it, if he or she doesn't already know.

Beware of healthy-sounding foods like yogurt, which in restaurants, is usually neither low fat nor sugar-free, and granola, which is the "fattiest" cereal under the rising morning sun.

Sandwiches

Sandwiches can be lean or mean. At home, most of us make a sandwich with a teaspoon of mayonnaise per slice of bread, but restaurants often slather 1 to 1½ *tablespoons* of mayo on their sandwiches. (One tablespoon of mayonnaise contains 100 calories and 11 grams of fat).

What goes between the bread makes a big difference too. Here are some good and bad choices.

Low-Fat Sandwich Filling

Beef brisket
Extra lean corned beef
Extra lean pastrami
Lean ham
Roasted chicken breast
Roasted turkey breast
Skinless grilled chicken breast
Veggie or soy burger

High-Fat Sandwich Fillings

Cheese
Chicken salad with mayo
Cold cuts
Egg salad with mayo
Fried fish
Hamburgers
Salami
Tuna salad with mayo

Several of the choices in the low-fat sandwich list above are standard on Subways menus in addition to salads. A 6-inch ham submarine has a moderate 360 calories and 45 grams carbohydrate.

Last but not least, portion size is important. Even if your diabetic friend orders a sandwich with turkey breast and lean roast beef, if it's a 12-inch submarine sandwich or 3-inch tall "deli monster" it's probably large enough to feed two people. Perhaps you could agree to share.

Salads and Salad Bars

Salads can be a low-fat meal or side dish that supplies a large portion of vitamins and fiber-rich foods, or they can be loaded with fat. Worse, many times people who eat a salad for lunch feel so virtuous that they go overboard at dinner, sure that they have some calories in their "bank."

Here are just two examples of salads that are *not* low fat:

Chef's salad (2 cups)   800 calories and 65 grams of fat
With cheese, boiled eggs
roast beef, ham, and turkey
roll with a creamy dressing

Salad Bar Salad (2 cups)   900 calories and 70 grams of fat
With bacon bits, sunflower
seeds, egg yolks, olives,
creamy pasta, potato salad,
and bleu cheese dressing

Either one of these salads has more calories than a double bacon cheeseburger with a regular order of fries! Salad dressing alone can make a salad a high-fat food. The amount of dressing in a ladle at a normal salad bar *holds 6 tablespoons*, which alone can equal the fat and calories of a Big Mac. The salads above were calculated to have 4 tablespoons of dressing, or 300 calories' worth. That's still a lot of fat for something as "unspecial" as salad dressing.

Here's what to *skip* to keep a salad low in saturated fat and/or calories:

Bacon bits	Macaroni salad
Cheese	Olives
Cold cuts	Potato salad
Croutons	Regular salad dressing
Egg Yolks	Seeds
Fruit and Jello in	
whipped cream	

Fried Chicken And Steak

What you should be looking for are places where you and your relative or friend with diabetes can get low-fat, low cholesterol dishes with generous portions of fruits and vegetables. Two eateries where you're not likely to find these choices in abundance are fried chicken restaurants and steakhouses that advertise extra-large portions. In fact, the beef served in many restaurants is USDA Prime–the highest in fat and calories. If there is no alternative to ordering beef, at least have a very small portion (doggie-bag the rest), and order it well done so that some of fat drips off.

You know that fried chicken is high in fat. There is a crispy version that is even greasier. One regular breast is 276 calories with 17 grams of fat. The extra-crispy version has 350 calories and 21 grams of fat. KFC now has a grilled breast with only 180 calories and 4 grams fat. But what to order with that? The side dishes that are traditionally served with fried chicken are better avoided. That includes the coleslaw, fries, sugary baked beans, and onion rings. The best choices as far as low fat goes are corn on the cob and mashed potatoes without gravy.

Again, you don't control the voice of your friend or relative with diabetes and he or she may order the dreaded crispy chicken. You will have to just bite your tongue when "You shouldn't have that!" threatens to escape from your lips. What you might do, however, is mention, in a low-key way, that you just learned that the extra-crispy chicken has more fat than the regular kind. Try being amazed and glad you found out and offer this valuable nutrition fact to your friend or relative as a gift, not a condemnation.

Vegetarian

Vegetarian restaurants can be healthy or not. It depends on whether they go heavy on cream sauces, cheese and nuts to make up for the meat they leave out. They also frequently serve huge muffins, which they bill as healthy because they are made from whole grains and "without sugar," though they are frequently full of fat and honey (or some other hyped "natural" sweetener). The sweeteners that cane and beets produce are just as natural as the sweetener bees produce, and all three raise blood sugar. "Natural" does not mean "healthy." Remember that lard is 100% "natural," but no one is recommending that you consider it healthy.

Seafood

Seafood restaurants usually have a good variety of low-fat protein. Try to avoid anything fried, breaded, dipped in batter, or served in a creamy sauce, such as lobster Newburg or thermidor. Tartar sauce and mayonnaise-based dill sauces should be used sparingly, while lemon juice can be used lavishly.

Good cooking methods to choose from are grilled, roasted, steamed, or stir-fired.

Pass on the Cajun blackened fish–it is dipped in melted butter then fried.

French

French restaurants may offer both high-fat choices and healthier dishes. It depends largely on the specialty of the house.

French restaurants that specialize in food from the north of France tend toward dishes with organ meats, paté, goose, sausage, lard, creamy sauces, quiche and croissants. These are high in saturated fat and cholesterol.

Restaurants with food based on southern France's cuisine are more likely to use seafood, vegetables, wine and small amounts of olive oil. Bouillabaisse, coq au vin, and salade Nicoise would be good choices.

Even if you can't find a southern French restaurant, you may be able to get food prepared as you and your friend or family member with diabetes prefer and stay within your fat budget. The staffs in French or continental restaurants seem to be more accustomed to fussy eaters, so requests to serve the sauce on the side or to cook without butter are accepted with aplomb. Also, the portion sizes are usually not so large as to lead one to overeat.

One caution–pastry carts are very tempting. It's best not to let one be brought to your table. "An ounce of prevention . . ."

Italian

Like French cuisine, Italian food varies greatly by region. The northern provinces tend to use more cream and meat. The southern areas, especially Sicily, go more heavily to tomato sauce.

In general, avoid pasta in butter, cheese, oil, cream, pancetta, or pesto sauce. Also avoid sausage, salami, cheese and bread drenched in olive oil or butter (garlic bread).

Good choices are tomato-based pasta sauces such a marinara, light red, vegetable, and red seafood. Order veal picata, chicken cacciatore, shrimp scampi sautéed in wine, or pizza with vegetable toppings–double the tomato sauce and halve the cheese.

By avoiding the rich foods and mentioning your healthier eating goals, you may inspire and give added weight to what your dining partner has surely heard before but may have thought was "too hard" for "regular people."

You can even get your diabetic dining partner in the mood for the healthier choices by raving about them when you propose the restaurant. Say something like, "Let's go to Roma's Ristorante. I hear it has great atmosphere and they have a marvelous chicken cacciatore. And I know how much you like chicken."

Making Sense Of The Menu

This brings us to the issue of how to find out exactly what is in the "pasta primavera" or the "trout almondine" and how to get it modified.

Ask Questions !

You or your family member or friend with diabetes must ask the server questions. Pasta primavera may *sound* healthy, but if those noodles and vegetables are bound together with a cheese, cream and butter sauce it's a high calorie artery-clogger. You need to learn what's in "mystery" dishes. If the order taker doesn't know, expect him or her to disappear into the kitchen and find out. Don't settle for "I *think* that's made with skim milk" or "That dish probably has pineapple juice, not corn syrup." Beware, also, of the "yes" person who just wants you to finish ordering and will say anything to speed up the process.

This is a great time for you to take the active role as questioner. If you ask for your own knowledge, your friend will not be made to feel different, and you will both get the information.

Request Substitutions

Not only do you sometimes need to know what's in a dish and how it's prepared, you may want to make substitutions. But what if your friend or family member with diabetes is shy, and before the waiter came to take the order, he or she said, "It's too bad that comes with French fries, I'm trying to cut down on fried foods." You know she'd like to skip the potatoes, so you, as the bolder one, can do the asking for her. This can be done in a way that does not single her out as different. For example, you can ask, "Can the fish be grilled without butter and served with lemon instead of almond butter sauce?" Or, "Could tomato slices be substituted for the French fries?" Or, "Can that be made with an egg substitute?"

Getting food cooked differently or ordering items on the side is much easier than it used to be. Even the fast food chains will frequently make it "your way," an accommodation that was unheard of not long ago.

Making Good Menu Changes

Here are some ordering tips to cut down on temptation and set a great example for your dining partner with diabetes:

1. Ask for a doggy bag when the food is served and "bag" whatever is not part of a sane portion *before* you start eating.

2. If doggy bagging is not an elegant option (such as at a banquet), sprinkle gobs of pepper on the forbidden food or portion, to render it inedible and free you from later pangs of temptation.

I got this tip from a woman who attended political dinners. It kept her from nibbling the pushed aside food during boring speeches.

3. Forget the usual appetizer, entrée, soup, salad, and dessert combination. Try a shrimp cocktail with a baked potato (sour cream and butter on the side), or salad and dessert, or half a melon and soup. This way you won't be eating a lot of food that just happens to come with that entrée and that you figure you've paid for, so you eat it. The a la carte/side dish method is also often cheaper than the full dinner plus extras.

4. Beware of menus that try to direct you to a safe choice. Often there is an infamous "Dieter's Special" that consists of a 6 to 8-ounce fried hamburger patty with a scoop of high-fat (creamed) cottage cheese accompanied by canned fruit in heavy syrup. It has about 700 calories and more than 40 grams of fat.

The much healthier "dieter's special" that I would recommend is a turkey breast sandwich on whole wheat or sourdough bread, with the mayo on the side. Almost anything is better than chips or fries, but the best substitutes would be tomato slices or a green salad with low-cal dressing, lemon juice or vinegar.

5. Pass up foods that are described using any of these words:

Almondine	Escalloped	Salad (if it means
Au fromage	Fried	mayonnaise is an in-
Au gratin	Gravy	gredient, as in tuna,
Au lait	Hollandaise	chicken, macaroni sal-
Basted	In cheese sauce	ad, cole slaw, etc.)
Breaded	In its own gravy	Sauce
Creamed/creamy	Marinated	Sauteed
Crispy	Pan-fried	Stuffed

6. Try to choose dishes that are described by these words:

Baked	Grilled	Steamed
Boiled	Lean	Skinless
Broiled	Roasted	Stir-fried

7. Condiments loaded with fats or sugar include:

Cranberry sauce	Tartar sauce
Barbeque sauce	Sour cream
Mayonnaise	Teriyaki sauce
Salad dressing	

You should be able to shock and amaze your audience by telling them that, ladle for ladle, salad dressing (except for low-fat versions) has more calories than hot fudge sauce. You could even add that you read that if diet dressing is not available, the next best choice is a small portion of a runny, non-creamy dressing (such as Italian or vinagrette) since most of those end up at the bottom of the salad bowl.

Another option is to have the dressing on the side, dip your fork into the dressing, and then stab some salad with the anointed fork. No chance of getting too much dressing that way but every bite will have some dressing taste.

8. Instead of mayonnaise, tartar sauce, and oily salad dressings, use low fat or fat free condiments such as:

Chili peppers
Cocktail sauce*

Horseradish
Ketchup*
Lemon juice
Mustard
Pickles
Salsa
Soy sauce (caution high in sodium)
Tabasco sauce
Taco sauce*
Vinegar
Worcestershire sauce

*These have some sugar and should be limited to a total of 2 to 3 tablespoons a day to still be considered a "free food."

9. Carry your own favorite diet salad dressing, diet maple syrup, jelly, chilies, or whatever will make staying within you goals more palatable. (Individual packets of diabetic products are available at restaurant supply stores and by mail order.)

My husband carries his own artificial sweetener because he prefers it to the brand usually available. In truth, we often carry a lot more than that. If we know there will not be a low-fat salad dressing, we bring our own. If he plans on ordering a particular sandwich, he brings his hot chili peppers. His instant coffee is less strong than restaurant coffee, so he brings that too, asks and pays for tea, gives the tea bag to me to take home, and just uses the pot of hot water. It is not difficult to have the best of both worlds–the variety and service of dining out *with* some of the comforts of home.

10. Soup is a great way to start a meal. Studies have shown that the calories in soup (not *cream* of anything, though) are a bargain because we tend to eat less of the rest of the meal.

Other good appetizers are fresh vegetables and salsa, seafood cocktail, marinated vegetables, and seviche. Ones to avoid include nachos, guacamole, deep fried mozzarella sticks, egg rolls and buffalo wings.

If no one else will order the seviche or marinated vegetables, be the adventurous one and by sharing, maybe introduce someone else (hopefully you-know-who) to a healthier alternative.

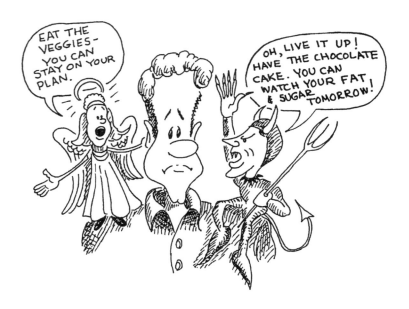

Be Loyal To Restaurants That Listen

Eating at a particular restaurant regularly makes requests for special preparation or substitutions easier and more likely to be honored. Valued customers can usually write their own menu selections *and* get a smile.

Remember that the restaurant wants your business, so whatever you need to take care of yourselves–whether that is information about ingredients and preparation or substitutions–will probably be provided. Sometimes you'll meet an uncooperative server or manager. Fortunately, in my experience, these are the rare exceptions but they do happen, and it helps to have an alternate selection or even a different restaurant in mind in case you can't get what you need. I've probably encountered half a dozen in many years of restaurant eating.

I once tried to order pizza with double tomato sauce and no cheese. The proprietor said that was too complicated for her cook to prepare. I left. It was easy to leave because I was with my husband, who supports my efforts to control my fat and cholesterol. I wonder if I would have left, though, if I'd been with someone that had decided that this pizza place was "it" and had been unsympathetic or reluctant to leave.

Smoke-filled restaurants and bars are best avoided too. Experts estimate that just 20 minutes of breathing smoke-filled air makes a non-smoker's platelets almost as "sticky" as the platelets of pack-a-day smokers–and therefore more likely to form clots that could cause a heart attack or stroke. Diabetics are at high risk for heart attacks and strokes, and, even if you believe you're not, it seems kinder to protect the more vulnerable people in your group.

There are times when being with our friends seems more important than being good to ourselves. Don't force your friends to make that choice.

Your Help Is Valuable

You and Lloyd's colleague Susan (from our opening story) now know how important meal timing and avoiding too much alcohol can be to helping Lloyd stay safe. You can explain to others that Lloyd *has* to eat between 6:00 and 7:00 P.M. not because he's a picky guy, but because his mealtime has to match his insulin.

When Susan learns more about diabetes, she can steer the group to eating within Lloyd's timetable and can choose a restaurant that offers many choices of foods low in cholesterol, fat, calories and sugar.

One way to head people toward choosing restaurants with the healthiest foods is to name three restaurants you know that serve healthy dishes and let the group choose from among the three.

> People seldom improve when they have no
> other model but themselves to copy after.
> Oliver Goldsmith

Why the emphasis on your choosing more foods that are low in fat, sugar and salt and high in fiber? (1) For your own better health and (2) Because if you're only a *coach* and not a *player,* you risk seeming to be a nag. If you *join* the person, you can rejoice together at great "finds," such as sugar-free, nonfat frozen yogurt and an excellent 95% fat-free salad dressing. And you can sincerely commiserate at the still-need-to-be-improved dietetic foods like sugar-free maple syrup. You can kid about what each of you thinks the world needs a whole lot more than a good five-cent cigar. My vote is for a luscious, fat-free, sugar-free chocolate fudge—with nuts!

If you're sharing occasional snippets of information about low-fat eating, be enthusiastic, but don't preach. Your goal is to educate your dining partner(s) about healthy eating and perhaps convert a few other people—*eventually*. Rome was not built in a day, everyone does not have to look like Brad Pitt and Angelina Jolie or have a cholesterol of 150 next week but it sure would be nice if we all had a cholesterol of under 200 at our next physicals.

9

Low Blood Sugar:
When Sugar Is Medicine

There is one situation where your knowing what to do in a hurry might be vital. That's when someone with diabetes has low blood sugar, also called insulin reaction, insulin shock, or hypoglycemia. A blood sugar of 60 or less is considered low blood sugar.

What It Feels Like to Jo

"My mouth gets dry and my tongue feels thick. Rivers of perspiration run from my scalp and forehead. I get shaky and rubber-legged, somewhat disoriented, but 'something' kicks in and I'll grab three or four glucose tabs or glucose gel. When I first got diabetes, I followed the dietitian's orders and drank orange juice or ate three graham cracker squares. The problem with those orders was getting my hands to take orders from my brain, so sometimes the orange juice didn't make it to the quivering glass. After the juice, I would *try* to wait 20 minutes for results (as the dietician also told me to do), but the symptoms always got so much worse before they'd start to get better that I'd find myself tearing into a candy bar. Now I just start with glucose or hard candy. This works better for me.

"In public or when someone is at home with me, I sometimes suddenly begin talking a blue streak, stuttering and acting jumpy. My husband knows what this means, and he'll ask me if I could be 'sliding.' In my insanity, I get very provoked and will go into a snit or even pout. This isn't *me*.

Towards the end of the second piece of candy treatment, I'll understand what's going on and can at least express my appreciation for his efforts.

"When I get low blood sugar in a grocery store or church, I feel profound dread and embarrassment. There I am, fumbling with candy wrappers while people look at me suspiciously.

"At night I sometimes wake up freezing cold and soaking wet, having no idea of where I am. Instinct kicks in, I search for "warm," so my husband becomes alerted and starts squirting glucose gel into my mouth while I'm giving him a hard time. I try to get away from him and the stuff he's trying to put in my mouth. My brain is so vacant, I'm sure that he's the one with the problem, not me. Once he manages to break into that fog (he'll holler or shake me, get me to sit up if he can), I'll very grudgingly cooperate.

"After I get past the worst by eating the glucose tabs or gel, I know I have to eat something more substantial to keep my blood sugar up, but the all-over sick feeling doesn't lend itself to appetite. I force myself to eat anyway.

"I feel wiped out physically, as though I've climbed Everest. I'm weak as a kitten and can barely lift my arms, walk, or sit upright. This can persist for hours.

"At night I may fall back to sleep, but I don't rest and in the morning I wake up feeling truly awful."

The Morning After

Jo's experience of feeling achy and unrested in the morning is shared by many people with diabetes. Even when they haven't awakened and been fed candy or glucose, their blood sugar in the morning may read in the 400s (normal is around 80 to 120 mg/dl). That's because their own emergency blood sugar supply from the liver has finally "kicked-in" to deal with the low blood sugar–too late to prevent the symptoms and a lot more than ideal or the reading wouldn't be 400. It can take half the day to bring this high a blood sugar back into the normal range.

Wondering Why It Happened

Jo's husband lovingly "grills" her about what could have caused her low blood sugar. Did she forget her bedtime snack? Did she take too much insulin? Did she remember to compensate for her exercise in the afternoon? Even when there's no one else that asks piercing questions, the person with diabetes asks them and feels guilty. He or she "must" have done something wrong to have caused this. Feeling guilty is not helpful. But asking questions to try to prevent a future low blood sugar caused by similar conditions *is* useful.

You as a helper need to remember that although most low (and high) blood sugar episodes can be prevented by good diabetes management, not all of them can. A perfect blood sugar is not possible without a cooperative pancreas.

What Could Cause a Low Blood Sugar

From the questions that Jo's husband asks her when probing for the cause of her latest low blood sugar, you can see that the usual ones have to do with food, medication, and exercise. Specifically, a meal that's too small, has little carbohydrate, that's late, or worse, skipped, is a frequent cause of low blood sugar. For people who take insulin or some kinds of pills, food has to be eaten close to when the medicine is at its peak of action.

That's why it's a very bad idea to take insulin and then get behind the wheel to drive to a restaurant. It's dangerous to drive when the last meal's food is long gone while there's a lot of insulin in the blood (either from an earlier injection or from pills that stimulate the pancreas). Lots of things could happen that would delay getting to the restaurant or delay getting served that could be at least embarrassing, at worst tragic.

Another cause of low blood sugar is taking too much insulin or oral medication. That could be because too much was drawn up in the syringe. Or it could have been injected into a thigh just before exercising so the insulin was absorbed more quickly than expected. Also, sometimes people need less insulin than they used to because they have lost some weight.

Exercise is the last of the common contributors to a low. Actually, it's not *too much* exercise that causes the low blood sugar, but the fact that the exercise wasn't compensated for by either reducing the insulin (before or afterwards), or increasing food (before, during, or afterwards). Diabetes and strenuous exercise are not incompatible, but like so many things about diabetes, even normal activities have to be planned.

Robert Polhill, an insulin-requiring diabetic, who was held hostage in Lebanon for 39 months, had about 400 low blood sugar reactions during that time. Many of his lows happened because his captors would insist he perform some unscheduled exercise like cleaning the room, sometimes with little or nothing to eat that day. The only treatment provided for low blood sugar was to drink some of the cola the guards grudgingly provided for that purpose.

Twice he didn't feel the low blood sugar soon enough and passed out. The other hostages managed to drizzle enough cola down his throat to bring him out of shock. This was extremely risky since he could have inhaled the cola while he was unconscious, but in this situation there was no other option. Thank goodness it worked.

So the three most common causes of low blood sugar are too little food, too much insulin, or more exercise than anticipated. There is a fourth cause, alcohol. Alcohol is such an important issue for the person with diabetes that it deserves a section of its own.

Alcohol and Low Blood Sugar

When a person with diabetes drinks alcohol, blood sugar can get too low. This is because when anyone–diabetics and non-diabetics alike–drink alcohol, the liver stops doing one of its most important jobs, which is to release stored sugar when needed. Whenever we go several hours without food, our liver supplies us with sugar to tide us over until our next meal. But when we drink alcohol, the liver only processes the alcohol and stops doing other tasks.

So alcohol, without food to keep the blood sugar up, is potentially dangerous for someone with diabetes. A single glass of wine with dinner is not dangerous, however, because the food in the meal will supply enough sugar to keep the blood sugar from getting too low, so the reserve supply in the liver will not be needed. The point is that alcohol can be safely consumed only in moderation (one or, at most, two drinks), and only with a meal.

Each of these equal 1 drink and have equivalent amounts of alcohol:

> 4 ounces of wine
> 12 ounces beer
> 1½ ounces liquor

Another serious safety issue is that it's difficult for the person with diabetes and for his or her friends to tell whether the person is tipsy or experiencing low blood sugar. Symptoms of a low include confusion, poor coordination, anger, and slurred speech. Is this person drunk? Would you know whether to put this person to bed or to treat him or her for low blood sugar? Probably not. And the person with diabetes would be too confused to tell you.

This is why moderation is not a word used lightly when drinking and diabetes are discussed. For example, in the case of a person with slurred speech, or any other symptom shared by both low blood sugar and alcohol excess, the recommendation is to try to get some juice and/or food into him or her and have someone spend the night checking the person every half hour for excessive sweating, tremors, or coma in case the blood sugar gets dangerously low. If that helper can check blood sugar with a meter, even better. If symptoms occur or blood sugar gets to 60, and the person can't eat or drink safely the helper should call for emergency help.

Early Symptoms of Low Blood Sugar

The early symptoms of low blood sugar are the same ones (though less severe and shorter) you or anyone may have felt when afraid or angry. They occur when adrenaline is pumped into the blood stream to prepare you for "fight or flight." It's a reaction to something your body thinks is an emergency. And since the body perceives low blood sugar as an emergency, it may feel and look very much like fear or anger. The symptoms are:

Sweatiness	Lightheadedness
Shakiness	Headache
Nervousness	Hunger
Irritability	Heart palpitations

Irritability and Low Blood Sugar

The symptom most family members think they can recognize, as a sign of low blood sugar is irritability.

At the first hint of testiness, they will say things like, "Don't you think you better have some juice? Your blood sugar must be low." This almost universally makes people with diabetes angry. I used to be puzzled by this because I figured if I were in that situation, I would rather someone think I was having a low blood sugar than think that I was a grouch. But this is not how people with diabetes see this. Here are some of their comments.

> "Ask me what is bothering me to determine if I'm really upset or if a low blood sugar is controlling my emotions."

> "Leave me alone unless I'm showing obvious symptoms and am not in control of what I'm doing."

> "Just remember everyone has a bad day now and then. Don't assume it's from diabetes."

Another reason for not jumping to the conclusion that irritability is due to low blood sugar is that irritability can mean just the opposite. The following is a common complaint:

> "Learn the symptoms of both high and low blood sugar and know how to deal with each, as needed. I get crabby when my blood sugar is *high*."

People with diabetes have all the emotions other people have. Sometimes they have something to be irritated about.

Also, the same symptoms that alert you to a possible low blood sugar could be the result of some other emergency. Even if you eliminate anger and fear, a heart attack or shock could be to blame. Keeping an open mind could mean catching a serious condition early.

Treatment

If the symptoms are caused by low blood sugar, eating something with sugar is the "cure." Surprised? Maybe you thought people with diabetes are allergic to sugar and always have to avoid it. Not so. A low blood sugar is an emergency situation that must be corrected, and sugar does the job.

If the person with diabetes is aware of the symptoms, he or she will probably reach into a pocket for glucose tablets, or get a regular (non-diet) soft drink or some juice. Now is *not* the time for the usual sugar-free soda—the person needs sugar and needs it quickly! One of the following treatments for low blood sugar is generally recommended:

> 1/2 cup fruit juice or non-diet soda
> 6–7 Lifesavers (about ½ a roll)
> 3-4 Glucose Tablets (check package–give enough to equal 15 or 16 grams carbohydrate)
> 1 tube oral glucose gel (a tube with 15 grams carbohydrate)
> 1 tablespoon honey
> 1 tablespoon sugar

What works quickest is glucose tablets or gel (glucose starts working in two minutes). Next speediest is a sugary liquid such as non-diet soda or fruit juice. It only takes 1/2 cup (4 ounces) to do the job. *The goal is to correct the low blood sugar and bring it back to normal.*

Years ago the treatment for low blood sugar was a humongous glass of orange juice with spoonfuls of sugar stirred in. That must have kept blood sugar from dropping again for a very long time. Sadly, It also shot it through the roof. In those days, however, you couldn't test someone's blood just anytime, so no one knew what that huge glass of juice did to the blood sugar. Now we know better.

A low blood sugar reaction is also not the best time for a candy bar. For example, a chocolate bar is about 50% fat. That fat actually slows down the sugar, which needs to get from the digestive system into the blood. So give glucose tablets or gel, if available. If not, some hard candy such as Lifesavers works well.

Back to your role as helper in this low blood sugar event: with the early symptoms listed above, your only job will be to fetch and carry if the person with diabetes is alert enough to ask for your help. But if the low blood sugar goes untreated until it gets much lower, a whole new set of physical signs can appear and you may need to do more.

The human body is a wonderful organism with many emergency backup systems. For example, there are several hormones that *raise* blood sugar. Glucagon, adrenalin, and growth hormone are just three and only one to *lower* it (insulin). That's to protect brain cells. If the blood sugar gets so low that it results in starved brain cells, it is a catastrophe for the body.

The first warning is the set of symptoms that are early signs of a low blood sugar: the sweating, nervousness, and so forth. They are indications that adrenaline is working to make the liver release its emergency supply of stored sugar. Unfortunately, there is not an inexhaustible supply, especially in people who have recently had several lows, so sometimes you, the helper, must do some or all of the correcting.

Symptoms of More Advanced Low Blood Sugar

Later symptoms of low blood sugar are due to brain cells being starved for glucose. They include the following:

> Confusion
> Slurred speech
> Lack of coordination
> Anger

Someone with these symptoms urgently needs your help. The confusion alone may prevent the person with diabetes from knowing what he or she needs to do. *You* must know and take steps.

What do you think a police officer would think if he pulled someone over with these symptoms? If you guessed, "the driver is drunk," you're probably right.

After stopping someone for erratic driving a police officer doesn't often think of diabetes, sometimes with tragic results. People have died in drunk tanks because the police thought they just needed to sleep it off when what they needed was sugar, or in extreme cases, medical help.

Treatment for More Advanced Low Blood Sugar

The treatment is still sugar. If the person is conscious, you can give 1/2 cup of non-diet soda or fruit juice in small sips or offer glucose or hard candy. Any of these things is okay unless the person has passed out.

Symptoms of Severe Low Blood Sugar

A low blood sugar that is not corrected may continue to get lower. The brain cells become starved for glucose, and they stop functioning. The symptoms of severe low blood sugar are:

Convulsions
Loss of consciousness
Death

Treatment for Severe Low Blood Sugar

You must never pour something into an unconscious person's mouth (unless medical care is far away and you have no other option). He or she could inhale the liquid or food and choke. It wouldn't get into the stomach, but into the lungs. If glucagon (more on glucagon follows) is available and you know how to use it, this would be a good time to get busy and do it. If not, call 911 or get the person to an emergency room right away.

Calling for Help

In this time of scarce medical resources, it's very important to be as efficient and accurate as possible when you deal with the call screener at the emergency dispatch switchboard.

The person you talk to first has to understand or be convinced that what you're reporting is a real emergency. He or she will probably pull it out of your eventually–but you can effectively cut to the chase and speed your friend's treatment by saying something like:

"My close friend (or whatever your relationship is) has lost consciousness, has diabetes, and is very likely suffering a low blood sugar emergency."

Using Glucagon

When someone is unconscious or having a seizure that you think might be due to low blood sugar, call for emergency help. The paramedics will assess the person and, likely inject some glucose into a vein.

If emergency help is not nearby, it's helpful to have glucagon (pronounced glue-ka-gon) on hand and to know how to use it. The person with diabetes should plan ahead, especially for a camping trip or other situation away from quick professional help.

Most people with diabetes who have had a serious low blood sugar are OK with a call to paramedics when necessary. However, one woman I remember well had another opinion.

M.B. had had type 1 for 30 years. Her low blood sugars came on fast, so she was a veteran in handling them and had trained her family how to help her when she couldn't fix them herself in time. She was adamant that they *not* call paramedics. When her husband or children had done this in the past, the folks in her small town talked about her ambulance team visits for days. Those busybodies said things like, "After so many years with diabetes, you'd think she'd have learned how to take care of herself by now."

One time a paramedic blabbed and M.B. found out when a woman in the supermarket said, "I heard the rescue team was out at your house last week. Dave (one of the paramedics) said you had a really cute black bra on." Clearly Dave needs to keep his mouth shut.

So you can see why M.B. might prefer that her family handle it.

An injection of glucagon is necessary only if the person cannot eat or drink because he or she is unconscious or having a seizure. It is rarely needed, but when it is, it is *very* needed.

There is nothing difficult about giving a glucagon injection. It can be given in the front of a thigh, or in the upper outer arm, or anywhere you have seen the person with diabetes take insulin (such as in the abdomen). You won't do any harm, and you might do a tremendous amount of good.

If you are extremely nervous about whether this will work, call for the paramedics and then give the shot. That way you know that if you don't do it just right, your backup is on the way, but you won't be letting the low blood sugar get worse.

The only tricky part of giving glucagon is mixing it up. It usually comes in a plastic box that includes a syringe containing liquid and a bottle with powder. The powder is the glucagon. It's in a dry form so it can be stored longer. You have to add liquid to make it injectable.

The liquid in a glucagon kit is in the syringe that comes with the powder. Take off the needle cap and inject all of the liquid into the bottle. Swirl gently to mix. Then pull back on the plunger to draw out the glucagon liquid. For a child, take out only half the liquid. For an adult, take it all out. Don't worry that if you give too much, you will overdose the person. Glucagon is not a medicine that needs to be precisely measured the way insulin does.

Take your thumb off the plunger, if that's where it is, hold the syringe by the barrel (the long part), and push the needle quickly into the arm (or wherever you decide to inject). Now put the thumb of the hand holding the syringe on the plunger and push in the fluid.

Occasionally someone will vomit after getting glucagon, so turn the person on his or her side so no stomach contents get inhaled. (Vomiting may also occur with low blood sugar–it's not always the glucagon's fault.).

Usually the person can be roused in 5 to 10 minutes–almost always within 15 minutes. Give 1/2 cup of juice or non-diet soda in sips or 1 tablespoon of sugar in 1/2 cup water as soon as he or can swallow safely after waking up.

If you have never given a glucagon injection before, you may be scared at the thought. Jo's husband is, and he's grateful that he has never had to use it. Still, he and Jo[1] are glad it's there, just in case.

You can rehearse for the day you might have to use the kit by walking through the steps without actually mixing or giving the glucagon. Know where the kit is. Look at the bottle and syringe. Leave the cap on the needle and pretend you are injecting the solution and so forth. Even pretend to give the injection to your friend or family member with the needle cap still on. Or, better yet, if the person takes insulin, offer to give the person an insulin injection at their usual time once or twice. You will have a chance to get over the scariest part at a time when the "injectee" is able to give instructions. You will feel much better about the real thing after any trial run.

---

[2]Jo has frequent low blood sugars because her pancreas was removed due to severe pancreatitis. Without a pancreas, she has no beta cells to make insulin and no alpha cells to make glucagon. Also, because of her surgery, she can't accurately predict when her food will leave her stomach and the glucose will start entering her blood, so it's hard to get her food and insulin in sync.

Practice is a big help. M.B.'s seven-year old son was alone with his mom one day when she sank to the floor unconscious. He had seen his dad and older sisters give glucagon lots of times so he grabbed the syringe in the kit and gave his mom a shot. Unfortunately, he didn't mix the liquid in the syringe with the powdered glucagon. When she didn't wake up in 5 minutes, as she usually did, he called 911. She got the help she needed and he never forgot that mixing step again.

Interestingly, although you don't need a prescription to buy some insulins, you do to buy glucagon. If your family member or friend takes insulin, needs help to fix low blood sugar occasionally, and does not have a glucagon kit for each place he or she spends a lot of time, encourage the person to ask the doctor for a prescription. It will just take a phone call to the doctor and a phone call and trip to the pharmacy.

The best place to store glucagon is in the refrigerator. It doesn't really need to be kept that cold (anything under 90° F. is safe) but it's an easy place to find it. You probably will never need to use the glucagon, so it will eventually expire. If there is a kit around the house or your colleague's office, ask to see the expiration date. It may need replacing. If it does, you can use the expired kit to practice actually mixing up the solution and injecting it into an orange before you throw it all away. Be sure to dispose of the needle as is mandated in your state. Some states require only that you break off the needle and put it in a crush-proof container; others want the needle and syringe placed in a Sharps container (a specially marked disposal box) and taken to a medical waste dump. Nowadays in this age of AIDS, custodians and garbage collectors get understandably upset when they get stuck with a hypodermic needle.

When Should You Call For Help If Someone is Unconscious?

When to call 911 depends. It depends on how familiar you are with your friend's, loved one's, or colleague's low blood sugar events. It depends on how long it would take emergency help to get to you, it depends on your own confidence in dealing with this emergency, and it depends on whether you saw the person lose unconscious or discovered him and don't know how long he has been out.

Let's look at the worst case scenario first. If you discovered the person unconscious and don't know how to test his blood sugar, call for emergency help immediately. If glucagon is available and you know how to give it, do that. If you don't have glucagon and you're too far away for help to get to you in 10 minutes and you can get the unconscious person into your car, drive him to the closest emergency room.

If you don't have glucagon, some sources recommend rubbing glucose gel, honey, or corn syrup on the inside of the cheek. Maybe enough will be absorbed to raise blood sugar a bit. The problem is that some of that syrupy stuff could be inhaled–a substantial risk. If he rouses enough to safely sip a sugary beverage, or suck glucose tabs give the appropriate amount of those or one of the other things that raise blood sugar.

If you saw the person lose consciousness, you may have a little more time. But how much is debatable. Some people faint when their blood sugar is 45, others can be as low as 15. Clearly, the one with a blood sugar of 15 has a very small window of time for you to get that blood sugar up. You need to act quickly–call 911 first and then give glucagon. The emergency response operator will help you decide what other options are best. At least, he or she knows how long it will take the paramedics to get to you.

If you test and the person's blood sugar is at least 45 you have a choice. Either give glucagon, wait 10 minutes to see if the person rouses, and then call for emergency help or call first and then give glucagon.

Some of the decision making is easier if you know the person's usual recovery from a low blood sugar. In the story about M.R., her son only waited 5 minutes before calling 911 because that was the time it usually took for his mom to wake up after getting glucagon.

Lastly, it depends on what the person with diabetes has said he or she prefers. It's a preference, not the law, though. You don't have to respect his wishes if you don't want to feel responsible for a possibly bad outcome. The person may not die, but low blood sugar can damage brain cells. Remember, there is no charge for the emergency team to come to where the person with diabetes is. And if he quickly revives, you can call the emergency operator back and cancel the help. Emergency teams tell me this happens in a multitude of situations when what looked serious, turns out to be no big deal.

What To Do When

If the person:	Do this:
Is irritable	Ask what is wrong.
Is shaky or sweaty	Offer to bring soda (*not sugar free*), juice, or candy
Is confused, uncoor-dinated, or has slurred speech	Give ½ cup soda, juice, glucose, or other sugar.
Is unconscious and you know how to inject glucagon	Prepare glucagon, inject, and turn on side in case of vomiting. Give soda or juice when conscious.
Is unconscious and you cannot inject glucagon	Call paramedics or take person to an emergency room.
Is unconscious, you can't inject glucagon, and there's no phone or transportation near.	Put glucose gel, honey, or syrup between gums and cheeks and stroke to en-courage swallowing. (Some authorities are afraid that even thick substances can get in an airway, but if no other option is available you need to do *something*.)

How Common Is Serious Low Blood Sugar?

Clearly, low blood sugar is not to be taken lightly. The good news, however, is that low blood sugar events that require help are not everyday events (except for people with unusual conditions like Jo).

Recent studies have reported that as few as 4% and at most 25% of insulin-treated people have one or more episodes of low blood sugar a year that require the help of someone else.

What To Do If The Person Doesn't Regain Consciousness

The patient may be in a coma from severe hyperglycemia (high blood sugar) or may have suffered a heart attack or stroke or a medical problem other than low blood sugar. In such a case, the patient will not respond to glucagon and requires immediate medical attention.

How to Be Sure It's a Low Blood Sugar

Fortunately, you no longer need to guess whether blood sugar is low or high if you know how to take a blood glucose reading with a meter. Below 60 is considered a low blood sugar and should be corrected. A blood sugar of 60 to 70 could need correcting soon–test again in fifteen minutes. A reading of 70 to 120 is in the safe normal range.

If you can't check the blood sugar, the safest rule is that if the person cannot get his or her own juice or sugar because of sudden confusion or lack of coordination, you should assume it's a low blood sugar and treat it. That's because a high blood sugar usually takes several hours, or even days, to become serious, while a low is serious *NOW*.

For example: say you follow the guideline above and give somebody one of the foods or fluids that have 15 grams of carbo-hydrate. If their blood sugar was 200 and that food raised it to 250, would that kill him? Absolutely not. Everyone with diabetes has had a blood sugar that high, and likely even higher.

But what if it was 50 and you did nothing and it went down to zero. That would be fatal. So the rule again is, if you aren't sure, err on the side of giving something to *raise* their blood sugar level.

After the Low Blood Sugar Is Corrected

Glucose and sugar work quickly, and that's why we use them to raise low blood sugar. However, they also wear off quickly–in about 30 minutes. The person recovering from low blood sugar will need something more substantial to keep the blood sugar from falling again.

A good snack would be:

1/2 sandwich (meat, cheese, or peanut butter)
or
a 6-8 oz light yogurt
or
1 oz cheese with 4-6 whole grain crackers
or
8-oz. glass milk

Or if the next meal is due soon, don't wait–serve it now.

A low blood sugar doesn't have to be frightening. Just know how your friend or family member's behavior changes when his or her blood sugar is out of control and do what is indicated.

Folks with diabetes tell me that their friends and family generally do the right thing when they have low blood sugar. Only about 30% say someone *once* should have done something differently and not one said he or she was put in danger because of a mistake.

Helpers Sometimes Do Too Much

The most common mistake in low blood sugar episodes is for helpers to overreact. Some relatives yell and blame. Other people tend to panic. Untrained friends and colleagues are prone to call an ambulance even when the person is conscious and says he or she is really all right and is recovering.

One Swedish exchange student said his American friends insisted on taking him to an emergency room despite his protests. He finally let them, just so they'd learn he was really okay. However, he wasn't used to our medical care costs in the U.S. He says the shock of the $700 hospital bill for a blood test, sandwich, and a five-minute chat with an ER doctor came a lot closer to killing him than the low blood sugar had.

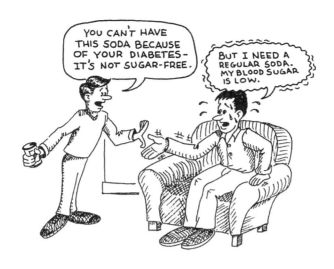

Professionals Sometimes Do Too Little

There is no guarantee that just because someone is a nurse, doctor, or paramedic, he or she will always make the best decision the first time.

Kira tells of a time when she was 16 and was driving long after she should have had her dinner (she was trying to lose weight by skipping a meal). She passed out and smashed into a parked car. Her only injury was that she hit her mouth on the steering wheel so she was able to give her home phone number to a witness. Her mother wasn't home but her sister was and rushed to the scene of the accident.

The police arrived before her sister, so Kira told them, "I have diabetes, I have low blood sugar." But the police officer kept asking, "What kind of drugs are you on?" In her confusion, when she looked in the rearview mirror and saw blood trickling from the side of her mouth, Kira said she was a vampire which only reinforced the officer's and the newly arrived paramedics' belief that she was on drugs. Her sister came during all this, pointed to Kira's Medic Alert bracelet, and asked for glucose, but all they wanted to know was, "What kind of drugs is she on?"

Kira was then taken to an emergency room, where the staff refused to give her anything to eat or drink because they needed to check her blood for drugs. Meanwhile her blood sugar was getting

151

lower and lower. Finally Kira's mother arrived, yelled at a nurse, and at last succeeded in getting her some juice.

These professionals all forgot the first rule of helping a confused or unconscious person you know has diabetes. *When in doubt, treat the person for a low blood sugar.* It will do little harm to give glucose tablets or juice if the person can swallow, or a shot of glucagon, if he or she can't. And if there's no improvement, other causes for the condition can *then* be considered.

The moral of this story is that you can do much better than that police officer, those paramedics, or that ER staff. You can check for a medical I.D. bracelet, insist that top priority be given to what it says, and you can yell like that mom for juice or get it yourself.

Medical I.D. Is A Good Idea

A medical ID bracelet or necklace pendant can be invaluable in getting help in a low blood sugar emergency. The well-known symbol of the Caduceus (a staff with two snakes wound around it) is internationally recognized as a designation for medical information. It gets people's attention and "speaks" for the diabetic when he or she can't. The word "Diabetes" engraved on the back tells people who know anything about diabetes and low blood sugar that when that person is confused or unconscious, the best thing to do is to call for medical help or (if help is not available quickly) get some form of sugar into them.

But which is best, a bracelet or a pendant? To get the answer I called the chief paramedics in three counties in Oregon. Each one said, "It doesn't matter, we look for both kinds." What all three added without any prompting from me was, "ID cards don't help us. We don't look in people's wallets."

A wallet card might be of some help once someone gets to an ER and the staff looks for info on next of kin and insurance, but if you want your friend or loved one to have a better chance of getting quick help–help that might make a trip to the ER unnecessary, encourage them to get some medical ID.

Some pharmacies sell basic bracelets or pendants for about $7.00. Another source is jewelry companies that advertise in diabetes magazines and on-line. Their products start at about $15. Regular retail jewelry stores also sell medical I.D. jewelry.

Another option is Medic Alert, a good choice for someone with a complicated medical condition. In addition to supplying ID jewelry, etc., Medic Alert relays stored vital medical information provided by the client to emergency personnel. The patient's file includes: medical conditions, medications, contact person, physician, etc. Medic Alert staff can be contacted in an emergency by calling the 24-hour toll-free number engraved on the ID tag. There is a yearly charge for this service.

Although Kira's bracelet didn't get the help she needed from the police, paramedics, or even the ER staff, in the vast majority of cases, medical I.D.s get the message across.

And thank goodness, there is usually good backup. There are people like you who now know what to do and are ready to do it.

10

High Blood Sugar: From Flu to ICU

Martha's Lesson

Martha's flu started with a headache, fever, and muscle aches. The next day she felt worse, called in sick, and stayed home. She tested her blood sugar (it was a little high, but not alarmingly so), took her usual morning insulin, fixed herself a bowl of canned soup, and spent the morning sipping a two-liter bottle of sugar-free soda.

In the afternoon Martha felt worse and went to bed for a nap. When she awoke it was dark. She hadn't eaten lunch but her stomach was upset, so she didn't want even soup. She was afraid that if she took her evening insulin without eating, her blood sugar would get too low so she just took another bottle of sugar-free soda to the bedroom and went back to bed. She didn't check her blood sugar because she wasn't eating anything, so how could it be high? And anyway, she was just too tired.

Martha had to get up twice during the night to urinate, which was unusual for her, but she figured that with all the soda she was drinking, that was to be expected.

The next morning Martha felt truly awful. She felt nauseated, her mouth was dry, and she was barely able to drag herself to the bathroom for what seemed the hundredth time. She did take her blood sugar, because she wasn't sure if she needed to take insulin since she couldn't bear the thought of eating. Her blood sugar was 486 (more than four times normal!). Martha called her doctor. Her doctor did not tell her to take two aspirins and call him in the morning. He told her she needed to get to the hospital right away, and if she didn't have anyone who could drive her, he'd call an ambulance. Martha called her sister, who got her to the hospital within an hour.

When Martha got to the emergency room, a nurse took her blood sugar. This time it was 502, Martha was breathing rapidly, she felt and looked flushed, and her tongue and lips felt as parched as a desert. A urine test showed ketones, and a blood test showed that her blood had become acidic. Diagnosis: ketoacidosis.

Martha was so dehydrated that she needed fluids by vein to replace what she'd lost in all those trips to the bathroom. She also needed salts and minerals. What she needed most of all was insulin. Ketoacidosis is caused by a severe shortage of insulin. Martha spent a day in intensive care getting intravenous fluids with insulin, plus salts and minerals to replace what she'd lost. Her blood sugar was taken hourly and all her urine was tested for ketones.

Her sister spent the day in the waiting room worrying.

The next day Martha was better and was transferred to a bed on the regular diabetes floor. Her doctor and the nurse diabetes educator gave Martha a refresher course on what to do anytime she's sick. Martha had a lot of questions for the nurse. Here are Martha's questions and the nurse's answers:

Why did my blood sugar get high even though I wasn't eating anything?

Sugar doesn't come just from food you eat. It can come either from the liver's stored glucose or from sugar the liver can make from protein in muscle tissue. So even though you knew you weren't taking in any sugar in food, you were getting a hefty supply from your liver.

Why did my liver "think" I needed more sugar?

Your body was fighting off a flu infection and needed extra energy to handle the stress of your illness. Your liver will do the same thing with any major stress like surgery, a heart attack or a stroke. Emotional stress, and even good news can bring on a release of sugar. One young woman told me she never had a high blood sugar with ketones until the day she found out she was finally pregnant.

Even if you hadn't been sick but needed extra energy, a low insulin level would have signaled the liver that it needed to give up some of its stored glucose. That's one of the ways the body tries to keep an even blood sugar between meals.

I guess I shouldn't have stopped taking my insulin then, right?

Right. You still needed insulin to get sugar into the cells, but none was available. When the sugar started accumulating in your blood, your kidneys tried to flush it out.

But I drank lots of fluids as you're supposed to when you're sick.

Yes, you did. That was good strategy, and it might have been enough for someone who didn't have a shortage of insulin and very high blood sugar.

I know I'm in the hospital for ketoacidosis and not just dehydration. Why did I get ketoacidosis?

When your cells couldn't get enough sugar to function, the body tried to use an alternate fuel supply–it used stored fat. The trouble with using fat is that it releases ketones (end products of fat metabolism) that makes the blood acidic. You felt nauseated and started breathing more quickly, both as a result of ketones. Your body needed insulin, fluids, and food to function properly.

But I felt sick to my stomach. I tried soup, but when I got sicker I didn't think I could keep any food down.

Soup was a good idea. Another food that seems to be tolerated when a person feels nauseated is saltine crackers. Ask any woman who ever had morning sickness what she was able to keep down, and you'll soon have a list of foods for sick days.

If even soup and crackers are out, you still need some calories, especially some carbohydrates to balance the insulin. Fifteen grams every one or two hours is recommended. Here is a list of some foods that have 15 grams of carbohydrate:

1/2 cup Jell-O (*not* sugar free)	1/2 cup apple juice
6 or 7 Lifesaver candies	1/2 cup orange juice
6 saltine crackers	3-4 glucose tablets
8 animal crackers	1 cup Gatorade
3 graham crackers	1 cup milk
1 slice toast	1/2 cup ice cream

1/2 cup cereal	1/2 cup fruit yogurt
1/2 cup soda (not sugar-free)	tea with 3 teaspoons sugar

If you can't drink a glass of juice all at once, sip it slowly so that you get 1/2 cup down every hour. Some people find sucking a regular Popsicle (again, *not* sugar free), works well; it melts so slowly that even an upset stomach can handle it.

It doesn't sound as if 1/2 cup of fluid an hour is enough when you're sick.

You're absolutely right. It isn't enough. You still need to drink at least 3/4-1 cup (6-8 ounces) an hour of sugar-free liquid to keep yourself hydrated.

Is that all I need to do: Eat, drink and take my insulin?

No, you need to check your blood sugar at least four times a day when you're sick. If it's over 240, test your urine for ketones.[2] If the test shows even slightly positive two separate times, call your doctor. Even if you don't have ketones, if your blood sugar is over 240 at two different times, call your doctor.

It's possible that the doctor can keep you out of the hospital by suggesting an adjustment in insulin, if it's done early enough.

Another thing that a doctor can do is prescribe something to counteract the nausea so you can keep eating and drinking enough to stay out of trouble.

This sounds like a lot of work for someone who feels terrible and just wants to sleep.

It is, and that's why it would be best if you weren't alone when you're sick. It's very helpful to have someone bring you fluids, remind you to check your blood sugar or do it for you, and call the doctor if you get worse or don't improve in 24 hours.

---

[2] Strips for testing ketones can be bought without a prescription at a drug store. Foil wrapped strips keep about 2 years before they expire.

At the very least, ask someone to phone you every four hours to remind you to check your blood sugar, drink, eat, take your temperature, and assess if you're confused.

Ketoacidosis can be deadly if not treated in time.

What kinds of things should my helper call my doctor about?

You or your helper should call if you:

Have vomiting, diarrhea, or stomach pain.

Have not been able to take fluids and keep them down for four hours.

Have a fever over 101° F. for more than 24 hours.

Have a blood glucose level over 240 twice.[3]

Have ketones in urine twice.

Have a breath with a fruity, sweetish, or acetone odor.

Have lost 5 pounds or more within 24 hours.

Martha went home the next day with a pamphlet on sick day management. Her sister made her promise to call her or *someone* the next time she was sick. She said giving Martha soup and Jell-O was better than wringing her hands in a hospital waiting room any day!

Who usually gets ketoacidosis?

There are three common situations when ketoacidosis occurs. The first is in people who don't know they have diabetes. The second is when insulin is not taken, and third is when an infection or other illness causes the liver to release sugar.

1. People who don't know they have diabetes

Ketoacidosis is rare in someone who produces insulin, so the people most at risk are those with type 1 diabetes. About a quarter of people newly diagnosed with type 1 have ketoacidosis. When John was diagnosed, he did not have ketoacidosis. He had frequent urination, thirst, hunger, and weight loss, which are all symptoms of high

---

[3] There may not be ketones in the urine of someone with very high blood sugar if they have type 2 diabetes. They can still become very dehydrated and develop a potentially fatal condition called hyperosmotic coma.

blood sugar. He had some ketones in his urine (ketonuria), but he had not yet gotten to the point of ketoacidosis.

Kira did have ketoacidosis by the time she was diagnosed. She had all the symptoms John had, plus vomiting and dehydration.

Sarah, who was 65 years old when she was diagnosed, had a mild case of ketoacidosis, although her diabetes turned out to be type 2. She had been so thirsty because of her not-yet-discovered diabetes that in the days before she was hospitalized, she drank quarts of juice. The vast amounts of sugar in all that juice, combined with her already insufficient insulin production, caused her to produce ketones.

Sarah recovered so quickly that her doctor discontinued her insulin and switched her to pills when she was well enough to leave the hospital.

2. People who reduce or omit their insulin dose

Reducing or omitting an insulin dose is the most frequent preventable cause of ketoacidosis.

Sometimes the reasons seem sensible, as they did for Martha, but it's just not a good idea to guess and assume that insulin should be stopped. The doctor should be in on the decision and it should be based on blood sugar readings.

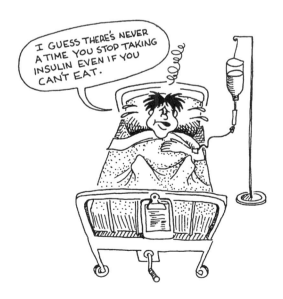

3. People with infections

Respiratory, urinary, and intestinal infections are the most common infections. Martha had the flu which was enough to raise her blood sugar and start the whole cycle of ketoacidosis and dehydration.

Next September, when the influenza vaccine again becomes available, Martha should get a flu shot. It will reduce her chances of getting the flu by 80%. The flu vaccine is recommended for everyone with diabetes over six months of age. It is considered safe for pregnant women. It's a lot safer than getting the flu during pregnancy, which could harm mother and fetus.

Even those with kidney, heart, or lung disease should be vaccinated. The downside is a sore arm. Martha will tell you that a shot beats tubes in your veins in the intensive care unit any day.

Pneumonia vaccine is also recommended for anyone older than two with diabetes. A second injection is recommended after 65.

Tetanus, although not common, is worth getting vaccinated against. It's a nasty disease that occurs almost exclusively in persons who are unvaccinated or inadequately immunized. The CDC recommends that adults get a booster every 10 years.

Why does ketoacidosis get out of hand?

The symptoms of ketoacidosis are frequently ignored because they could be due to a dozen different conditions. Flu frequently causes an upset stomach, so people like Martha don't think of ketoacidosis. Some even get a tender and swollen abdomen, which suggests gas or an inflamed appendix or other problems instead of ketoacidosis.

Finally, low blood sugar is so tiring and scary that people with diabetes work hard to prevent it. They learn that insulin must be balanced with food, so when they can't eat, they think omitting their insulin is a good idea. They forget that food is not the only source of sugar, that the liver can supply it too.

What if ketoacidosis doesn't get treated in time?

Martha was lucky that she called her doctor while she still could. She might have gotten so weak and sick that she could have gone to sleep and never awakened again. That sleep could have become a diabetic coma. She might still have gotten treatment in time to be saved, but only if someone had found her before she became one of the up to 10% treated for ketoacidosis who die of irreversible coma or one of the other fatal conditions caused by dehydration and related problems.

Another High Blood Sugar Emergency Condition

Hyperosmolar, hyperglycemic nonketotic syndrome (HHNS) is a serious condition most often seen in older people. HHNS sometimes occurs in those with undiagnosed type 2 diabetes and in those with diagnosed type 2 after long periods of increasingly elevated blood sugar. HNNS is usually brought on by a recent surgery, infection, stroke, heart attack, or other illness.

As with ketoacidosis, people with HHNS suffer from profound dehydration as a result of severe high blood sugar (usually over 600) but do not have ketones.

Warning signs include: warm, dry skin that does not sweat, high fever, confusion, and hallucinations.

Many victims get high blood sugar, don't drink enough water, and gradually get too weak to ask for help. Sometimes a stroke leaves them helpless in their home.

If HHNS continues it can result in seizures, coma, and death.

How You Can Help

Nurses consider themselves "the patient's advocate." You, too, can be an advocate by looking out for your friend or family member's best interest. For the elderly, who live alone, this may mean calling once a day even when they are apparently well.

For someone you know is ill, call at least once a day, and visit if you can. Heat soup, help with blood sugar testing, or do whatever he or she will let you do.

You may be able to prevent someone with diabetes from jumping to the wrong conclusion (for example, thinking that their vomiting is from eating a bad piece of fish–instead of ketoacidosis), or from taking his or her illness too lightly and not testing often enough or not calling the doctor.

It's important, if you do visit, to take a good look at the person. In the case of someone with type 1, look for rapid breathing, a flushed face, drowsiness and slow reflexes. This could mean ketoacidosis. At the least, it means that it's time to test and call the doctor.

11

Complications Go From Head To Toe

Robert was 43 years old and had a huge infected sore on his swollen foot when he was admitted to our hospital. He had had a small blister on his foot a few days before, but it didn't hurt so he ignored it. The next day the blister looked red and ugly but he didn't have medical benefits with his job as a cook, so if he went to a doctor, he'd have to come up with the money for the visit out of his own pocket. On the fourth day the blister had grown into a large gaping sore and he couldn't get his shoe on his swollen foot. It still didn't hurt, but to work in a kitchen he was required to wear closed toe shoes so he had no choice–he had to see a doctor. The doctor took one look at his foot and ordered a blood test. His blood sugar was 430 mg/dl–the first clue Robert had that he had diabetes. The doctor admitted him to the hospital within an hour. Two days later it looked as if he might need an amputation. It took two operations and four weeks in the hospital to save his foot.

Complications Of The Feet And Legs

How did a blister turn into a huge sore and almost lead to an amputation? That's what can happen when even a painless sore gets infected. In someone who has had high blood sugar for some time, as Robert did, though he didn't know it, nerves get damaged. Sometimes affected feet tingle or ache. Often they have no sensation at all. This is not the blessing it might seem. Not feeling pain means not getting a message that something needs attention. Robert would have seen a doctor much sooner if that blister/sore had hurt as it should have.

Robert also had partially clogged arteries from cholesterol and other fats in his blood, so the body's infection fighters couldn't get to the injured tissues in the amounts needed.

High blood sugar provides a more favorable environment for infectious organisms to grow–lots of sugar is a banquet for germs. In addition, white blood cells don't fight infection as well when sugar stays in the blood and doesn't fuel those cells.

This combination of lack of sensation combined with poor circulation and decreased ability to fight germs is tough on feet.

While he recovered, Robert was given all the usual instructions about diabetes with special emphasis on foot care and a low-fat, low-cholesterol diabetes meal plan. Fortunately, he rarely drank alcohol, so he didn't need to be counseled about how alcohol aggravates nerve damage (neuropathy). The foot care precautions he learned included never going barefoot, preventing or quickly treating athlete's foot, inspecting feet every day for sores that he might not feel, not soaking feet, and not risking injury with "bathroom surgery" such as trimming corns with a razor blade.

Robert had some changes to make. He was about 30 pounds overweight, his cholesterol was 265 instead of under 200, and, of course, his blood sugar before he came into the hospital was high. But Robert left the hospital with a good understanding of diabetes management, his new diet, a blood glucose meter, and the motivation to never let a blister turn into a medical emergency again.

If this sounds too unbelievable, the lack of feeling that Robert experienced is not unusual.

I once attended a lecture on neuropathy by renowned neurologist (nerve specialist) Aaron Vinik, MD. He started by taking off his shoe and feeling around inside while he talked. He said, "I always check the shoes of someone with neuropathy. I'm mostly looking for worn linings and wrinkles and holes in insoles. But one day I felt something in the toe and pulled it out. It was a wristwatch. The patient was delighted. He said, 'Thanks, Doc, I've been looking for that for three weeks!'"

Objects in shoes can scratch, gouge, poke, and stab. Sometimes it's a lancet, sometimes a child's toy–the possibilities are endless.

What the doctor illustrated with his story is that people with diabetes need to check their shoes before putting them on.

Robert's complications are among those that people with diabetes worry about. We'll also discuss the tasks that are part of good diabetes care and preventing complications, why those tasks aren't easy, and some of the feelings that are associated with diabetes. You'll read about what to do and what to avoid to help your relative, friend, or co-worker with diabetes succeed.

Causes

Many diabetes complications, including Robert's, are due to some change in the blood vessels in the body caused by the disease. Since all cells rely on the blood vessels to bring them oxygen and food and remove waste products, any narrowing or damage that causes these transportation lines to work poorly means the cells they supply suffer and may die.

Kidney and Eye Disease In a Young Man

Danny was a patient on the diabetes floor at a hospital where I worked. He was 22 years old and had had type 1 diabetes for 13 years. He'd been admitted to the hospital because of an infection that raised his blood sugar dangerously high. One of the reasons the infection had gotten out of hand is that he couldn't test his blood sugar because he'd recently lost his remaining sight. His eye doctor wanted to continue with laser treatments on his eyes but for Danny, laser therapy had only worked for a while and he'd had enough disappointment with it. He felt continuing was useless. While he was in the hospital getting the infection treated, he learned how to use a special blood glucose meter with a speaker for the visually impaired.

Danny had been living alone until three months before, but his recent worsening sight had made that impossible so he moved back with his father. He was on the waiting list for rehabilitation classes at the Institute for the Blind, which he hoped would enable him to live independently again one day.

The next time I saw Danny he was back in the hospital, groggy and sicker than ever. There was a note in his chart about drug and alcohol abuse, and that he smoked a pack of cigarettes a day. But whatever the cause of his getting sick this time, Danny's kidneys were failing, and he was started on dialysis. He felt so sick that he didn't want to eat and he lost weight despite his nurses' best efforts to entice him with his favorite foods.

Danny probably suffered a stroke that affected his brain because he never completely regained his former alertness. Eventually he was transferred to a nursing home. Three times a week he was taken back to the hospital in a wheel chair for kidney dialysis.

We all felt terrible for Danny and his family, and we wished we could have done something to prevent the terrible consequences of his poorly managed diabetes. Diabetes educators and physicians frequently think that if they say just the right words they will provide the critical seed of motivation. Danny made some bad decisions when he was a rebellious teenager: major complications in someone as young as Danny almost always happen after years of being in very poor control. Certainly his smoking, a major contributor to strokes and kidney failure, didn't help.

Complications Of The Eyes

The blood vessels that supply cells in the eye are very tiny. When blood has a lot of sugar, it becomes thick and flows with difficulty. When thick blood is combined with high blood pressure (another frequent condition in diabetes), the tiny vessels in the eyes can bulge until they rupture. When that happens, the body tries to fix them by mending the break with scar tissue and by growing new blood vessels to supply the areas the ruptured vessels served. If no more thick, gooey blood were forced through the damaged vessels and the fragile new ones, and if the blood pressure could be reduced, there probably would be no more damage. But if high blood sugar and high blood pressure aren't corrected, more vessels will be damaged and more new ones formed. The scar tissue that is supposed to mend may instead grow under the retina of the eye and detach it from the back of the eye. Where this happens, the person sees a blank spot.

Laser treatments can often be successful in fastening the retina back into place. The same instrument can be used to seal off bleeding vessels.

If bleeding into the usually clear eyeball has been so great as to obstruct sight, the blood can be suctioned out with the liquid in the eyeball and be replaced with a clear substitute fluid.

These treatments have saved sight for thousands of people with diabetes. To be most effective, they must be started when damage is not too severe. That's why the American Diabetes Association recommends yearly eye examinations by an eye doctor who dilates the pupil with drops to examine the eye thoroughly.

In addition to yearly eye exams, the sources of the damage–high blood sugar and high blood pressure–*must* be controlled. This may require a strict low-fat/low-salt diabetes meal plan, appropriate exercise (no weight lifting, etc.), medication to lower the elevated blood pressure *and* blood sugar, plus blood tests.

This is why Danny's eye damage continued to progress; his blood sugar was not well controlled, it was too high too much of the time.

Using alcohol and drugs probably meant he paid less attention to diabetes management than he should have. He also smoked, which further constricted blood vessels all over his body, including those in his eyes.

The leaky blood vessels and detached retina described above are parts of a condition called retinopathy. It is one of the major causes of blindness in the United States, but it isn't the only eye condition brought on or worsened by diabetes.

Glaucoma is twice as common in the diabetic population and can result in reduced peripheral vision or even blindness. A gradual blockage of the normal outflow of fluid in the eye increases pressure inside the eye enough to damage the neurons in the optic nerve. If diagnosed early it can usually be effectively treated with eye drops, laser therapy, or surgery.

Lastly, a cloudy lens in the eye, called a cataract, is also more common in people with diabetes. Fortunately, a cataract is easily removed surgically and a plastic lens can be implanted that restores clear vision.

Kidney Disease

The causes of kidney disease (nephropathy) are very similar to the causes of retinopathy. Thick, sugary blood being forced under high pressure through delicate kidney blood vessels causes damage to the kidney.

The job of the kidney is to remove waste products from the blood as it flows through the kidney. If the blood is forced through at higher than normal pressure, it causes stretching in the kidney's blood vessels. Stretching causes collagen (a fibrous substance), to form a support network that eventually thickens the kidney walls. The result is a stiff kidney that filters poorly.

Treatment of kidney disease involves controlling high blood sugar with diet, exercise, and medications and high blood pressure with diet (low sodium), medications and, if needed, weight loss. In addition, a low-protein diet can help ease the blood vessel constriction that causes higher pressure inside the kidney. If protein in the diet is reduced at the first sign of kidney damage, along with the other treatments, damage can frequently be slowed, and perhaps the kidneys can continue to function adequately for the rest of the person's life.

Kidney damage doesn't have early symptoms that enable a person to know what's going on, so microalbumin urine tests that measure tiny amounts of protein in the urine, or a blood test for kidney function, should be ordered by the doctor at least once a year. This is another reason why physician visits are so important–to discover problems like kidney damage early enough for preventive measures to help.

If the kidneys lose their ability to filter enough waste products and get them out in urine, they build up in the blood, making the person feel very ill. The waste products then need to be removed by filtering the blood through a process called dialysis. The most common type of dialysis is done by inserting a needle into a large blood vessel in the arm and connecting it by a long tube to an artificial kidney machine. Blood is allowed to circulate through the machine for about three hours while nurses keep a check on the patient and the machine.

A second method of dialysis, called continuous ambulatory peritoneal dialysis (CAPD), uses the peritoneal cavity in the abdomen as a filter and collection place. It involves implanting a tube called a catheter in the abdomen through which a solution flows from a bag into the body. The solution stays in the abdominal cavity for several hours soaking up waste products that are usually removed from the blood by the kidneys and passed out of the body in the urine. In peritoneal dialysis, these waste products pass from the blood through the blood vessel walls inside the abdomen and collect in the dialysis fluid.

Every few hours, the fluid is allowed to drain out of the body back into the bag. This process is repeated several times with bags of new fluid, until the person's blood is cleansed of many of the waste products the kidneys can no longer remove.

Some people are able to do this kind of dialysis at home themselves or with the help of a family member. They can even go shopping or travel while doing their dialysis. Judy Curtis, in her book *Living with Diabetes Complications,* tells how her dialysis was so routine that she could do it in the car, at work, in airports, on trains, and even on an airliner.

Neither method of dialysis is pleasant. Being hooked up to an artificial kidney machine usually means going to a kidney center three times a week and lying on a recliner for three hours at a time. Because people whose kidneys don't work make little or no urine, any liquid they have had since their last dialysis treatment accumulates inside their bodies. When three days of fluid is removed in three hours it leaves people feeling exhausted; their body chemistry is altered suddenly and their blood pressure is usually low. They must also adhere to a strict diet without most fresh fruits or vegetables, dairy products, meat, beans, nuts, or salt, and very little coffee, water or other liquid–anything harmful to the body when it accumulates for days must be reduced or eliminated.

Although peritoneal dialysis doesn't require as restrictive a diet as regular dialysis since the removal of waste products is done daily, it has its own drawbacks, including the chance of an abdominal infection and backaches from walking around with all that fluid inside the abdomen while the treatment is going on.

Another type of peritoneal dialysis called continuous cycling peritoneal dialysis (CCPD) or automated peritoneal dialysis (APD) uses a machine which is programmed to exchange the dialysis fluid at periodic intervals during the night while sleeping. The machine is expensive and for some people an exchange is also needed during the day.

After months of dialysis, whether with an artificial kidney or peritoneal dialysis, many people opt for a kidney transplant. The five-year success rate is now around 80% if the kidney is from a closely matched living relative. But even a kidney from an unrelated donor (usually a cadaver) has a 70% success rate.

Dialysis costs around $44,000 a year, while a transplant costs about $55,000. Both are reimbursed by Medicare and insurance companies.

The drawbacks to kidney transplants are that about 20% of transplants don't succeed. In that case, a second is needed. And for those that succeed, the recipients must take drugs for the rest of their lives to prevent their immune system from rejecting the kidney. Anti-rejection medicines have side effects and are also very expensive (about $16,000 a year), though Medicare pays for them for the first three years. After that, the patient or insurance company must pick up the cost. Despite all these negatives, life is definitely more normal with a donor kidney than on dialysis.

Complications Of The Heart And Circulatory System

The same fatty deposits that shut off some of Robert's blood supply in his feet might have blocked an artery supplying some part of his heart. If that had happened, Robert could have had a heart attack. If an artery in his head had been blocked, he could have had a stroke. High blood pressure adds more strain to damaged, hardened blood vessels and makes a heart attack or stroke even more likely.

Heart disease and stroke are probably the least recognized complications of diabetes, and yet if you visit a cardiac care floor at a hospital and ask how many patients have diabetes, you'd be amazed. They often go together.

The risk for cardiovascular disease can be reduced with these steps:

- Don't smoke. Smoking constricts blood vessels, including those in the heart and brain.
- Control blood sugar. Aim for an A1c of less than 7%.
- Control blood fats (cholesterol and triglycerides) by eating a diet low in saturated fat and trans fats and by taking cholesterol lowering medications, if needed.
    LDL (bad) cholesterol should be less than 100 (less than 70 is recommended for those at higher risk).
    HDL (good) cholesterol should be 40 or more for men, 50 or more for women.
- Control blood pressure to under 130/80 (120/75 is better). Sometimes it takes four different blood pressure medicines *and* a low salt diet to get to a safe BP.
- Control weight. Excess weight around the waist is particularly risky.
    Men - waist measurement should be less than 40 inches (Asian men less than 34 inches)
    Women - waist measurement should be less than 35 inches (Asian women less than 31 inches)
- Be physically active at least 30 minutes each day
- Get assessed for sleep apnea (loud snoring and gaps in breathing while sleeping).

Signs and Symptoms of a Heart Attack

Most heart attacks are not the way Hollywood portrays them: sudden and intense. Typically, they come on slowly, with mild pain. The pain may even go away and return.

Chest pain is the most common symptom but pain or discomfort can also be felt in the neck, jaw, one or both arms, back or stomach.

Some people don't feel any pain. Instead, they may have shortness of breath, nausea, lightheadedness, anxiety, or a cold sweat.

Don't wait more than 5 minutes to call for emergency help.

Signs and Symptoms of a Stroke

Signs of a stroke include sudden numbness of face, arm, or leg, especially on one side of the body; sudden confusion; trouble speaking or understanding; sudden trouble seeing in one or both eyes; sudden trouble walking, dizziness, loss of balance or coordination; and sudden severe headache without a known reason.

Note the time the symptoms started. This could be important later in deciding on treatment.

Don't wait more than 5 minutes to call for emergency help.

Getting Help for Someone with Heart Attack or Stroke Symptoms

When someone has symptoms that could signal a heart attack or stroke, you have two choices: call for emergency help, or drive them to the hospital yourself.

You might be tempted to drive your friend or family member to the emergency room to save time. A recent study showed that people who drove themselves (egad!) or had a friend or family member drive them got there, on average, 8 minutes sooner than those who came in an ambulance. But, *the ones who came in an ambulance got treatment 23 minutes sooner!*

Besides, if the person went into cardiac arrest while you were driving, would you pull over and do CPR or drive faster? Neither of those choices is good. Leave the transport and treatment en route to the paramedics.

Misguided Avoidance of Medications: Fear of Side Effects

Cardiovascular disease prevention and treatment requires a lot of different medications. For blood pressure control, up to four different meds may be needed; for cholesterol two types; for blood sugar control up to three. And some of these need to be taken twice a day. That's a lot of medication. To many people it seems excessive or plain unnecessary.

170

I often hear people who are prescribed a medication say, "I told the doctor I wouldn't take it; I don't like medicines, they have side effects."

I understand what a nuisance side effects can be but here's another way of looking at that issue. Here's Ray's story:

Ray comes to my diabetes support group. In addition to type 2 diabetes, he has asthma. His asthma is so bad that he has to take prednisone (a steroid hormone) to keep his airways open.

The prednisone causes water retention so he now has to take a diuretic (water pill).

Three hours after he takes a prednisone pill his blood sugar shoots up to 400, so now Ray takes insulin to control his blood sugar.

The prednisone depresses his immune system (it's a drug they give to people who have had organ transplants to prevent rejection), so Ray gets sick more often.

Prednisone is hard on the stomach lining so he needs a medication for that.

Prednisone leaches calcium from the bones so now Ray has osteoporosis and uses a walker.

Finally, prednisone increases one's appetite–something Ray didn't need any help with.

After I tell that story, I usually ask the "medicine avoider," "Why would anyone take a medicine that causes all those nasty side effects?"

What I often see is a look of disgust, a shaking head and sometimes a muttered, "I sure wouldn't."

But there is a more important question than, "Does it have side effects?" The better question is, "Am I better off with it than without it?"

If your loved one or friend is nixing a medicine, has he asked himself that question? If it's a blood pressure medicine, for example, has he considered that there are serious "side effects" to high blood pressure, such as a stroke, eye damage, or kidney failure?

In Ray's case it's pretty clear that he needs prednisone *to breathe*. He tolerates the side effects and the extra pills and insulin he has to take, because he's better off with it than without it.

An unexpected story about a side effect comes from the famous neurologist. Dr. Vinik.

He'd prescribed a red pepper cream (Capsaicin) for a woman with neuropathy. One day, her husband came charging into his office followed by a flustered receptionist, saying, "I'm so sorry Dr. Vinik, I couldn't stop him."

The man lunged at Dr. Vinik, grabbed the lapels of his lab coat, and roared, "Are you the doctor who prescribed that pepper cream for my wife?"

Dr. V. says he remembers stammering, "Yesss."

"Why didn't you tell her to wash her hands before we had sex!?"

So maybe it *is* important to ask about side effects too.

Impotence

Impotence, also known as erectile dysfunction (ED) is the inability to get and keep an erection and have normal ejaculation. The penis requires a good blood supply and properly functioning nerves which can both be damaged by diabetes.

The conditions that contribute to the development of ED can be minimized with these recommended actions:

- Control blood sugar. Aim for an A1c of less than 7%.
- Control blood fats (cholesterol, etc.) by eating a diet low in saturated fat.
- Control weight. Excess body fat interferes with testosterone and contributes to high blood sugar.
- Exercise most days of the week. This improves circulation—*everywhere* in the body, helps normalize weight, blood sugar, blood fats, and mood.
- Get treated for depression. Depression can interfere with sexual function.
- Avoid or limit alcohol to no more than 2 drinks a day. Alcohol damages nerves and raises triglycerides (one of the blood fats).
- Quit smoking. Smoking constricts blood vessels and decreases nitric oxide levels needed to maintain an erection.

The doctor may prescribe an ED medication. They are about 50% less effective in men with diabetes but are worth a try unless there are medical contraindications. A blood test of testosterone level is also advisable.

172

A urologist can help with treatment and other options to manage ED. There are mechanical vacuum devices that can restore the ability to produce and maintain an erection. Penile suppositories and even a medication given by injection into the penis are options. A surgical implant is another possibility. Penile implants are expensive but over 80% of the men who get them report that they are satisfied.

I remember reading a letter in an advice column in which an impotent man wrote that his doctor had offered him the option of an implant. His wife did not share his enthusiasm, however. Her response was, "I'd rather have a new dining room set."

That brings me to the last option: counseling. Just because a man has a physical reason that affects his sexual performance doesn't mean he can't also be wracked with anxiety and have that anxiety worsen the situation. Relearning sexual skills and rediscovering intimacy with his wife could enrich them both, even if none of the other options works or is acceptable to them.

For more see Chapter 13, Sex, Love, and Diabetes.

Other Complications

There are dozens of other complications, varying from mild to severe, that are associated with diabetes. Most have nerve damage, clogged blood vessels, high blood pressure, or all three in common. Some lead to damaged joints, others result in stomach and intestinal problems. Women can have problem pregnancies.

You've seen the same recommendations listed again and again.

Escaping Complications

Not everyone with diabetes gets serious complications. Thousands of people have received the Joslin 50-year Medal. To earn this medal, the recipient must have lived over 50 years with type 1 diabetes. Close to 50% of Medalists appear to have escaped the serious eye, kidney and nerve complications that typically occur after 30 plus years of living with the disease—most of that time before blood glucose meters were available!

It probably helps to have good genes in addition to carefully managing one's diabetes. Since no one can choose ancestors, a person with diabetes must rely on *good management* to prevent complications. And good management requires lots of motivation and hard work.

Preventing Complications Is Not Easy

When we hear about the serious complications that can happen to people with diabetes, we tend to think, "If I had diabetes and I could go blind if I didn't take care of it, I would stay on my diet and do everything the doctor told me."

Part of your certainty that you would do everything may be due to an unrealistic idea of just what doing everything involves.

Here is a list of the daily tasks of a *perfect* patient who has type 2 diabetes (remember, they have it only a *little* easier than folks with type 1):

1. Test blood sugar at least once a day unless the doctor says it's okay to test less often.
2. Record all blood sugar results and times.
3. Record any unusual events, such as missed exercise, feeling ill, etc.
4. Take all medications as prescribed.
5. Eat meals at scheduled times.
6. Follow a prescribed meal plan.
7. Limit concentrated sweets.
8. Limit protein in diet (if recommended).
9. Eat low-saturated fat and low-cholesterol foods.
10. Follow a weight loss or weight maintenance diet.
11. Exercise six or seven days a week.
12. Test blood sugar before exercise and during and after exercise if it's vigorous or extended.
13. Inspect feet daily and apply lotion.
14. Carry glucose tablets or candy and other snacks if low blood sugar is possible.
15. Carry meter and other supplies to work, school and social events.

Above are just the daily tasks. Less frequent but also essential chores include the following:

1. See doctor in charge of diabetes care three to four times a year if no problems, otherwise more frequently.
2. See eye doctor at least once a year.
3. See podiatrist every three months if feet need special care for corns, calluses, thick nails, etc.
4. Consult with dietitian if diet needs changing.

5. Buy supplies.
6. Fill out insurance forms.
7. Attend lectures and support group meetings and read diabetes magazines to stay current and motivated.

You might have two reactions to those lists. Maybe you said, "Wow, I had no idea what was involved in diabetes self-management. I'll be more considerate and understanding now that I know." If this was your response, give yourself a pat on the back and read on for more details.

If you thought, "That really doesn't look so bad. Some of those things only take a few minutes," you're partly right about that too.

Time

The time needed for specific diabetes chores may or may not seem to be a lot. It depends largely on how the person with diabetes regards the list and what is already part of his or her lifestyle. For example, for a 50 year old lawyer who doesn't exercise and who comes home dead tired every night around 9:00, finding an hour for exercise can seem a huge burden. He may say to himself, "What's the use, I don't have the time or energy, so why even try?"

But for a person who never gave up exercise or who got back into the habit before being told exercise is an important part of diabetes treatment, it's like being told to keep breathing. "Nooooo problem." When asking a regular exerciser how long he spends on his diabetes management every day, he's likely to say 10 to 15 minutes.

At first I used to be alarmed by hearing "10 to 15 minutes." I'd think, "This person is not taking care of himself. He couldn't do everything he's supposed to do in less than half an hour." But he could, if he's only counting checking his blood sugar, taking insulin, recording both, and checking his feet after his shower. Those things are do-able in 10 to 15 minutes.

And the "eating correctly" part needn't take any longer either. Or more correctly, it doesn't take longer when it's part of an established routine. It's time consuming when a diet sheet has to be referred to or a nutrition book consulted, or a person is writing out a week of menus for a dietitian to check, or when a trip to the grocery store requires reading a dozen Nutrition Facts labels. While someone is learning the diet and new diabetes management, it can seem as if it's taking over every waking hour. If you remember back to when you were first learning to drive, you'll be able to relate. Didn't it seem that there were fifteen things you were supposed to do simultaneously? Your instructor barked, "Watch the rearview mirror, signal a turn, don't follow too closely, slow down, take your foot off the gas, and parallel park over there." You never thought you would be able to do it all without being nervous and stressed every minute. But if you've been driving for years, you know how automatic most of your moves have become.

That new-driver feeling comes back when diabetes is new or insulin has just been started, or a new meal plan is prescribed. A person feels swamped with pamphlets, cautions, and instructions from the physician, nurse, dietitian, or all three, and diabetes may again seem to require constant attention to details and to the clock.

People with diabetes give a range of from 10 minutes to 2 hours per day for their diabetes chores. From discussions with them in greater depth, I know that this reflects only in part how complicated their diabetes routine is. It is more likely an indication of what they're omitting because they consider it a normal task (exercise and fixing a meal) versus what they label as a strictly diabetes chore.

Caroline puts it this way, "I only spend about a total of 20 minutes a day, but I always must be aware of my blood sugar and how I feel 24 hours a day."

It's somewhat like going about your day while you try to remember the items you need to buy at the market later on. It means being aware of mealtimes and insulin or medication times plus feelings of tiredness, nervousness, or hunger that might mean a low blood sugar reaction.

Time is not the only thing people with diabetes need. These tasks involve motivation, planning, money, inconvenience, and/or discomfort. Some, like pricking a finger to get a blood sugar level, involve more than one.

Other Concerns

Many of these issues were discussed in detail in Chapters 4 and 5. But here is a quick re-cap of why people may not do *everything* they can to prevent complications.

It requires planning and record keeping. Blood sugar testing requires supplies and keeping track of blood sugar numbers, medication (especially insulin) dosages, and notes about illness, low blood sugar, etc.

It's expensive. Medications, test strips and other supplies, doctor visits, lab tests, diabetes magazines–it all adds up.

It's inconvenient and awkward to test and take insulin at work and in social situations. Postponing it can mean forgetting it.

It hurts. Not the insulin shots–those are usually painless. It's the fingersticks.

It's something *they* say I have to do. *They* nag about food, testing, everything.

It's frustrating. Even if I do everything right I can get high or low blood sugars. Sometimes I just want to give up.

If I know what my blood sugar is, I'll have to do something about it. That means interrupting what I'm doing at inconvenient times.

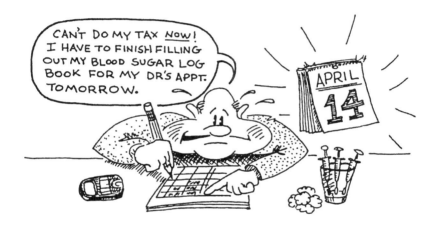

What Makes People Do Almost Everything They Should

You now know why diabetes management is difficult. So what keeps your friend or family member with diabetes doing any of these expensive, frustrating, time-consuming chores? People with diabetes I've talked with and who have answered my questionnaires, say that what usually keeps them on their diabetes program is, indeed, fear of complications. They may not do everything perfectly and consistently, though. The fear of a bad outcome just isn't enough to *always* overcome all the other demands on their time and resources.

Most people think it's the seriousness of the consequence that motivates someone to diligently follow a treatment. That may very

177

well follow with a surely fatal disease like some kinds of cancer. After the patient is convinced of the operation's necessity and agrees to have it, he has the operation, he goes for chemotherapy or radiation treatments, and eventually he's done with the whole thing. With diabetes there's never an end to the treatment, and it's the patient that does almost all the work, not the surgical team, chemotherapy nurses, or the technicians in radiology. Diabetes requires lifelong day-in and day-out discomfort, expense, food sacrifices and inconvenience. Motivation needs to be found again and again.

No matter how serious the possible outcome is, most of the time it is the number and difficulty of the tasks and adaptations that determine whether the person will follow the diabetes management plan or not.

Think of health routines you may or may not be following. If you're a woman, you probably go to the doctor for a yearly pap smear. But do you do a monthly self-exam of your breasts? If not, is it because you're not sure it's necessary? Or maybe you're not sure you know how to do it perfectly. Or you need to sign up for a class to learn how, but you don't have transportation, or it costs $15 and you're short this month. Or perhaps your doctor doesn't ask you if you do it and reward you with a "good work" when you say you have, so you think it can't be that important. In short, it's very easy for a physician to say, "You need to do this, it's important." But you know that the doing is much more complicated.

Another example is flossing your teeth. Do you do it every day? It's hard to remember to make that part of your bedtime or aftermeal routine, isn't it? If it is a habit you don't need to remember–it's automatic.

Diabetes management is like that. It's hard to make all those tasks habits, but once they are, they become second nature. That's one of the reasons this book stresses *helping the person with diabetes to stay on track and not break good habits*. It can be hard to get them back again once temptation has been tasted. Try to put yourself in the shoes of someone with diabetes: imagine a time when you made a list of New Year's resolutions. You were going to lose weight, quit smoking, or practice piano regularly, or something else that probably would be good for you. How many of those resolutions did you keep–for how long? Yes, it's tough changing old habits even when the goal is a worthy one.

Fortunately, other motivating factors can come into play when the burden of changing routine seems huge or the fear of complications seems less compelling and more remote. My patients also mention not wanting to feel tired or sick, the challenge of seeing how well they can do, accepting diabetes as something they just have to deal with, and wanting to be alive with loved ones. But these attitudes usually come with some experience and maturity.

Parents have an especially hard time instilling in their teens the motivation to eat sensibly, test, and take insulin on time. What seems to work best with this group is to emphasize how taking care of themselves can help them be and stay independent. Discussing goals and how good control can help realize these goals is also useful. *No one* can play well in sports or realize a dream of being a good *anything* if high or low blood sugars are sapping their energy and concentration. There has been a Miss America, and a number of top pro and Olympic athletes with type 1 diabetes. They've made it clear that *the discipline that made them great at what they do came, in part, from learning to take care of their diabetes.*

You can't do it for your child. You can provide the tools and offer help with working through problems without giving unsolicited advice. You can help your teenager see and understand himself or herself. But discovering the benefits of taking good care of oneself is ultimately a one-person job.

How Not To Help

Avoid saying, "You should . . ." or "You shouldn't. . ."
Avoid saying, "You never . . ." or "You always . . ."
Avoid saying, "You can't . . ." or "You must . . ."
Avoid judging.
Avoid nagging.
Avoid criticizing.

When you do any of these things, you sound like you're coming from a place of superiority. You think you know what's wrong and how it should be solved. However, unless you have a chronic disease that requires the work that diabetes does, admit that you don't *really* know what it's like. And even if you're right about what's wrong and how to solve the problem, the person may do the opposite rather than let you be proved correct.

Imagine the feelings of the 53 year old woman whose mother accused her of eating candy whenever her blood sugar was high.

179

Even if it were true, could she correct the problem without admitting that her mother was right? Would she *want* to prove her mother right? She'd be giving her mother proof that nagging works!

How much more effective it would have been if her mother had said, "I see your blood sugar is above the range you're trying to stay in. Is there anything I can do to help?" This shows respect for the person's feelings and a willingness to work this out *with* the person instead of having him or her *do it alone*.

Keep the long-term picture in mind. *Don't become the enemy in order to be right once*, or to hear the doctor side with you.

Now let's look on the positive side and see what you *can* do to help.

How You Can Help

1. *Describe, don't judge.* In the above example, the helper described the blood sugar as "above the range" but did not evaluate it as a "bad" blood sugar due to splurging. Or if she had noticed that her daughter had had cake that afternoon and maybe that was why her blood sugar was up, she could say (if it's true), "I noticed that you've been eating sweets this week. Do you feel under more stress than usual?"

2. *Be specific.* In the example above, the mother pinned down the behavior to this week. It makes it clear that there is some recent change that may have a specific cause, not just the person's "badness" or "laziness."

3. *Show empathy.* Imagine that your friend or family member has just told you about the time his or her diabetes was diagnosed. This is usually a milestone in a person's life, on a par with the birth of a baby–it changes one's whole life. An example of a pitying remark would be, "You poor thing." This makes the person think you see him or her as a helpless victim. A better, more empathetic response would be, "I had no idea that you went through all that." You could open up further communication, by asking, "Is having diabetes as difficult as you imagined it would be when your doctor told you the diagnosis?"

4. *Welcome positive changes.* This sounds as if it doesn't need mentioning. Of course you would applaud health-promoting

changes. Not necessarily from the bottom of your heart, though. You might see time at the gym as time stolen from you and the family. Or a support group could seem threatening because those people understand having diabetes in a way you never could. That understanding might mean bonding in a way you think you can't compete with.

Sometimes you can join the gym, too, or accompany your special someone to the support groups and learn. Or, if that's not possible, it would be best to accept and adjust. It is important, though, to recognize the resentment for the natural thing it is and grow from the experience.

5. *Help keep temptation away.* This could be as simple as not having foods high in fat and sugar around the house or office. It can mean choosing restaurants with healthy choices, or preparing low fat meals with fresh fruit for dessert. It could mean educating friends who put your family member or friend in situations where they are less likely to take care of themselves (like going out to drink every night after work).

When I ask people with diabetes what they wish friends, colleagues, and family members would do to make it easier to control their diabetes, they say, "Don't have stuff around that I can't eat." At one diabetes educator's meeting, when I asked that question, three dietitians simultaneously said, "Don't bring Oreos in the house." (At 53 calories, 7 grams carbohydrate, and 2 grams of fat each, an Oreo may not seem *so* bad but dietitians know that nobody stops at one). Even if your friend or loved one with diabetes resists the temptation, they are likely to say, if asked, that they feel bad when people eat sweets in front of them. If we care about someone, we don't want to be the cause of their sadness, do we?

How much of a sacrifice would it be to not have unhealthy food available? (After all, there are many other opportunities to eat junk.) I know a severe asthmatic whose husband and son go outdoors to smoke. I was also a guest at a Thanksgiving dinner where wine wasn't offered because one of the invited relatives was a recovering alcoholic.

You read how Pat's husband helped her by allowing her to banish the donuts. Pat tries to carry this a step further for other people. She helps out at a church where men's groups have meetings. The standard refreshments are huge platters of cookies. Pat suggested that maybe they could offer fruit instead of, or at least in addition to the cookies. She was hooted down by the refreshment committee, but she hasn't stopped trying. And I hope she doesn't. "Most of the men are overweight and could use a little less temptation," Pat added.

Rome wasn't built in a day, Pat's husband didn't sprout wings and a halo overnight, and maybe your family or group will need a little persistent bargaining.

For that social or office group, maybe just the *addition* of a healthy snack (like the fruit platter Pat suggested) would at least give some options to folks whose diet plan doesn't include cookies.

The next time your church, club, temple, or other group suggests an event with refreshments, how about suggesting a baking contest or pot luck with only low fat and/or low sugar foods? Try expending a little extra effort in making the low-fat, low-sugar treat look terrific. Fruit kind of takes care of itself with its great colors but other foods like fat-free muffins may need a cherry on top or decorative paper liners. Bring out the paper doilies and tiered cookie plates.

Another reason for keeping junk food out of sight is to reduce "pay backs." Pay backs happen when people deny themselves treats but later "reimburse" themselves.

For Martha it worked like this: yesterday she passed up the donuts at the office, the pie in the company cafeteria, the chocolates a colleague passed around the office, and the dessert on the pastry tray at dinner although she really *loves* éclairs. At home, as she was cleaning up the living room, she found a half-full bag of chocolate chip cookies her son had left on the sofa. She had denied herself four times that day. "That amount of sacrifice deserves a reward," she told herself, and down the hatch went five cookies. And she didn't even feel the guilt that splurging usually brings, because, from her point of view, she'd "earned" those cookies.

It needn't have happened, though. If Martha had had fewer temptations that required willpower to overcome, she might never have had her "cookie compensation" event. If you are a friend, fellow worker, husband, daughter, or son of someone like Martha, you can be a great help in keeping the total of her tempting moments to a minimum, thereby lessening "payback."

Part of keeping temptation away is to help the person with diabetes not feel different. It's hard to have to choose between being like everyone else and "being good." If no choice needs to be made, staying on one's diabetes management plan is easier.

6. *Be patient.* This refers to the times you have to wait for your friend to have a snack before you can start your bike ride, or times you have to eat earlier than you'd like because of his or her medication. It includes trotting off to get some juice when a low blood sugar hits. The more irritation you show, the guiltier your friend, co-worker or family member will feel and the worse you'll feel when you reflect on your impatience and lack of understanding. Again, recognize and accept your resentment as natural, but work on doing better next time. There's got to be at least one inconvenient trait you have that is irritating at times. There's satisfaction in doing good and being nice.

7. *Set a good example.* If you were considering losing weight, or switching to a low-fat, low-cholesterol diet, starting to exercise regularly, or quitting smoking, do it now and be a good example. You may be able to commiserate and praise each other. When one of you is ready to jump off the wagon, one can save the other. The roles will be reversed from time to time when weak moments come.

8. *Praise.* Finally, people with diabetes say praise from you, the people that are important to them, is a powerful force. Be sincere and recognize a positive effort or result. A "Good work on taking your blood sugar after dinner," or "I noticed that you exercised almost every day this week" is the kind of pat on the back that is likely to motivate the person you're applauding to test after dinner or to keep exercising regularly in the future.

12

Exercise: The Good,
the Bad, and the Ugly

The Hike That Went Terribly Wrong

Evan went on a weekend hike with a group of acquaintances. He was well prepared for the all day hike: in his backpack he had water, snacks, lunch, and his blood glucose meter. He even took along his insulin because he took a shot before dinner and sometimes the hikers didn't get back in time to eat at home– they stopped at a diner on the highway.

After they'd been hiking for awhile, Evan complained of feeling tired and sweaty but other people felt tired and sweaty too–after all, they *were* climbing. He apparently didn't consider that these were also symptoms of low blood sugar, so he didn't test or have a snack. As he plodded on, he used up more and more sugar. Eventually his blood sugar got so low that he passed out.

The others on the hike stood around trying to figure out how to help. One or two people knew he had diabetes so someone dug around in his backpack to see if there was something that would help. One "good Samaritan" found the insulin, and gave Evan a shot. Evan died on the trail.

My question to you is who is responsible for Evan's death?

Most people (including those with diabetes) answer that it was Evan. They say that he should have told people that he had diabetes, and what to do if he started acting differently (had glazed eyes, was unusually quiet *or* talkative), seemed more tired than usual, seemed sweaty and cold, etc.

Not knowing what to do, they chose the worst thing. If they had done nothing, his liver might have released enough emergency sugar to revive him. Then he could have eaten or had some juice.

Another option, would have been to trickle some juice into his mouth. This is very risky in an unconscious person but in this instance, far from medical help, it would have been better than doing nothing.

The worst choice was giving insulin because this drove his blood sugar even lower.

But why would anyone give someone a shot of insulin– a drug they clearly weren't familiar with? Because everyone knows that insulin has been life-saving for thousands of people with diabetes.

And most folks would never think of giving juice or candy because they believe that people with diabetes should avoid sugar.

This won't happen to an Evan you know, after you've read this chapter.

Exercise With Type 2 Diabetes

Remember Pat, the 57-year old schoolteacher with type 2 diabetes you met in the introduction? Pat needed to lose weight–at least 50 pounds. So far, she's lost 30 with a combination of diet and exercise. Her husband helped with both. Without his joining in her walking, Pat probably would have given up and been on insulin by now.

But she didn't give up because with his company, walking became a chance for them to get away from the phone and TV and share their day's experiences. They started walking three times a week after dinner and increased that to five or six times a week. When Pat had strengthened her leg muscles and lost a few pounds, she felt more energetic. That exercise bike in the corner of the bedroom that she'd been using as a clothes rack for the last year, looked interesting again. She started riding the bike on rainy days. She even watched some TV while she pedaled away. "It's impossible to rummage in the fridge while you are pedaling a bike," Pat says.

So eight months later, Pat had lost the weight, had almost normal blood sugar, and had reduced her diabetes medication. Her doctor didn't shake his head anymore at every office visit and threaten to start her on insulin.

Needing to lose weight, normalize her blood sugar, and wanting to stay off insulin were the reasons Pat got serious about exercise, but they're not why she keeps exercising. Now she walks and rides her bike because she feels more energetic and less stressed. Exercise no longer seems like work and it renews her belief that she can control her body.

Exercise With Type 1 Diabetes

For John who has type 1 diabetes, planning to go for a bike ride means, just that, planning. He doesn't just call up a buddy, jump on his bike, and ride to their meeting place. He often reduces his morning insulin dosage by a couple of units. Then he tests his blood sugar before the ride. His blood sugar at that time tells him if he needs a snack before he starts exercising. For example:

If the bicycling he'll do won't be strenuous (not uphill or very fast) and his blood sugar is less than 100mg/dl, he has half a sandwich with a glass of milk or a piece of fruit. If his blood sugar is between 100 and 180 he has just a piece of fruit or six saltine crackers. If the test reads 180 to 240, he doesn't eat a snack. For a reading over 300, he doesn't exercise.

It might seem strange that John doesn't exercise when his blood sugar is over 300. He needs to lower that blood sugar and exercise ordinarily does that. However, John doesn't have enough insulin available, if he did, his blood sugar would not have gotten over 300—the excess sugar would have left his blood and gone into the cells. If he goes ahead and exercises anyway, after a few minutes his muscles will send out signals that sugar is needed and his liver will try to help by releasing stored sugar. What will that stored sugar do to his blood sugar level? It will go up even more. Without enough insulin to move the sugar into the cells, it can't be used, so it accumulates.

So even though exercise *usually* lowers blood sugar, it doesn't if the blood sugar is already very high.

Once in a while, when it is quite a bit over 300, John drinks a lot of water and maybe takes a little fast-acting insulin. In 30 minutes or so, he re-tests. If it is below 300, he exercises. What can his friend do while this waiting is going on? He can keep John company and not act disappointed or disgruntled. Perhaps this is the kind of time the sage was talking about when he said, "Stop and smell the roses." Sometime ago, when his blood sugar was over 300, John and his friend relaxed under a tree and talked for an hour. The couple of times this has happened, they still had enough time to take their bike ride.

On days when John's blood sugar is not so high and they start out, his friend can help if John has a low blood sugar. This has never happened when they've only been riding for 45 minutes or so at a moderate pace. But when they are puffing up hills or making a day of it, John might run out of glucose if he doesn't snack every hour. He takes his meter with him and tests from time to time so he knows how much to eat.

If John forgets to snack or underestimates the amount of food he needs he might get the tiredness, shakiness, sweating and light-headedness that indicate a low blood sugar. If he knew it was low, it would be important to quickly take something containing sugar before he feels worse and becomes confused. The problem with these symptoms is that they can be normal responses to exercise that anyone can feel. Blood testing is the best way to differentiate between the two. You can't just rely on the diabetic's assurance that he is fine because when someone has a low blood sugar he often doesn't know it. Confusion may make him unclear about what's going on. Depending on your relationship, and the diabetic's willingness, you might want to learn how to test his or her blood sugar. The new meters are practically foolproof and the test takes only a minute or two from start to finish. It's okay to wait a couple of minutes for the time it takes to test before giving something to raise the blood sugar–but don't wait any longer. The usual remedy for low blood sugar is 1/2 cup of regular soda or juice. If your buddy has glucose tabs, give three or four. (See Chapter 9 for more on low blood sugar.)

Sometimes low blood sugar events happen long after the exercise is over. From 3 to 30 hours is the range. Experience helps teach the diabetic what exercise for what duration and at what intensity will lower blood sugar too much. There are steps he or she can take to compensate for that low. A bigger than usual snack at bedtime or a smaller than usual insulin dose is often recommended.

Despite the added inconveniences that exercise brings, there are so many advantages, that it's worth every extra finger stick.

Benefits Of Exercise

Can you name three reasons why exercise is good for everybody, including you?

Actually there are many more. Here are ten:

1. Exercise strengthens the heart. It does this by forcing the heart to work a bit harder. Exercise works on the heart muscle just as making an arm muscle work harder makes it stronger. A stronger

heart is capable of more forceful beats so that when extra work is asked of it, the heart muscle can increase its effort without straining.

2. Being able to exercise with some effort without undue straining means you'll feel more energetic in your everyday activities. Climbing a flight of stairs or mowing a lawn will be less tiring.

3. Weight loss is much more effective when diet is combined with exercise than with dieting alone. Exercise increases metabolism (the rate at which we use calories) and the size of muscles. Muscles need more energy than fat tissue, so bigger muscles use more calories even when they're not being exercised. Nice to imagine them using up calories even while the rest of you is asleep.

4. A better body shape is a bonus even if the scale shows no change. Muscle tissue weighs more than fat so even if weight stays the same, the replacement of fat pounds with muscle pounds, especially those on thighs and around the middle, means a slimmer shape.

5. For people with diabetes the effect that exercise has on blood fats (cholesterol and triglycerides) is extremely important. Exercise raises HDL (good) cholesterol, while it lowers LDL (bad) cholesterol and triglycerides. These effects lessen the risk for clogged arteries that can lead to stroke and heart attacks.

6. Exercise helps reduce the risk of strokes and heart attacks in another way: by lowering blood pressure. And that's not the only benefit; lower blood pressure lessens risk of damage to eyes and kidneys.

7. Weight bearing exercise is associated with increased bone density and reduces risk for osteoporosis.

8. Exercise, along with fluids and adequate dietary fiber, helps prevent constipation. Older people with weak abdominal and pelvic muscles may benefit the most, but it's good for everybody but the laxative manufacturers.

9. Last, but not least, for people with diabetes, exercise reduces blood sugar two ways. (1.) It increases insulin sensitivity by

increasing the number of insulin receptors on the body's cells. Since people with type 2 have a shortage of these receptors, having more can lower insulin requirements. (2.) Exercised muscles take sugar from the blood even after the exercise is over. It uses this sugar to replenish its reserve supply.

Sadly, not everyone takes full advantage of what exercise can do. Mr. H. didn't.

I usually ask folks in my diabetes classes to tell us what medications they take. One day Mr. H., a retired gentleman with type 2, surprised me when he said he unhappily took insulin every other day. I had never heard of someone doing that. He explained that he didn't need it on the days he swam laps at the community pool. Since he clearly didn't like taking insulin and swimming days gave him a reprieve, I asked him why he didn't swim every day. His answer? "Ah, it's too much trouble!"

Even if Mr. H. swam laps everyday, he might eventually still have had to take insulin everyday, but his story is a good reminder of how exercise can be a great ally in getting good blood sugar. Just one more reason for you to help your friend or family member to think of exercise not as "too much trouble" but enjoyable–if the exercise is the right kind for him or her *and* if you're along to make it social.

In someone with slightly to moderately elevated blood sugar, exercise has a proportionately greater blood sugar lowering benefit. Because the higher the blood sugar is (as long as it's no higher than 300), the more exercise will lower it. But for someone with diabetes, starting exercise with blood sugar in the normal range, lowering it further can be a problem. That's why snacks and blood sugar testing are such important parts of safe exercise.

10. Even if you don't have diabetes, exercise can be of great benefit to you. One study showed that men who exercised vigorously five or more times a week experienced a *42 % reduction in diabetes* compared with men who exercised less than once a week. Even exercising only once a week was demonstrated to reduce risk of developing diabetes by 23 to 33 %.

If you are overweight and have a family history of diabetes you can help yourself, while you help your diabetic relative or friend. Walk, swim, dance, whatever . . .

Other Benefits

Most of these benefits are long-term and some of them even require lab tests to confirm that exercise works. It's not always easy to stay motivated to do something that's good for you when you can't see any difference. Fortunately, exercise also produces almost immediate and positive effects that can make your diabetic relative or friend's and your day or night.

Exercise improves sleep patterns, mood, and the ability to deal with stress. And the only side effects are a little sweat and a rosy glow.

Risks Of Exercise

As wonderful as exercise is for almost everyone, there are some risks for all of the people some of the time and some of the people all of the time. For example:

1. A cardiovascular or respiratory condition may become evident with exercise. The usual symptom that signals a heart problem is chest pain. However, some people do not feel the pain that signals that the heart is not getting enough blood. Only when they exercise do they have other symptoms such as exceptional weakness and shortness of breath that tell them something is not right. People with diabetes are especially prone to this condition called "silent ischemia," because of damage to the nerves of their heart.

A pre-exercise evaluation by a physician should reveal any problems. He or she may recommend a stress test. That means an electrocardiogram (EKG) is taken while the person rides an exercise bike or uses a treadmill. This is much more reliable than an EKG taken while lying down. It shows how the heart reacts to exertion. Another way to assess heart function is by taking a 24-hour EKG. A small EKG machine called a Holter monitor is worn while the patient goes about his or her normal activity.

A physical examination before starting an exercise program is a must for anyone with:

a. Diabetes for more than 10 years;
b. Multiple cardiovascular disease risk factors any combination of high BP, excess weight, smoking and diabetes;
c. A sedentary lifestyle in one who is more than 35 years old;

d. Any known blood vessel disease or nerve damage. People with eye or kidney complications need to avoid exercise that can raise blood pressure and further damage the fragile vessels in these organs. Strenuous weight lifting is an example of a form of exercise that temporarily increases blood pressure.

2. Foot injuries or sores (blisters or worse) can happen to anyone even if he or she doesn't have diabetes. Preventing foot injuries and sores starts with wearing proper footwear. Well-fitting shoes that are s-l-o-w-l-y broken in, are a must. Anyone who is prone to blisters will find two-layer socks (sold in sporting goods stores) a help.

Before putting on socks and after taking them off, a smart person with diabetes checks his or her feet for sores, red spots and calluses.

Further, anyone with nerve damage or decreased circulation in their feet and legs needs to avoid activities that could cause injury. Soccer comes to mind; it's darn hard on shins. Going barefoot is also risky and should be kept to a minimum.

3. Hyperglycemia (high blood sugar) can worsen if blood sugar is more than 300 before exercise.

Despite a green light from the doctor, health problems might still occur during exercise. Here are some of the things to be on the lookout for in your exercise buddy:

- Difficulty breathing or breathlessness that continues longer than usual. This could indicate a heart problem or other condition.
- Pain, pressure, or aching in the chest, stomach, back, shoulder, neck, arm or jaw could be symptoms of a heart attack, as could nausea and anxiety.
- Joint pain lasting more than two hours is not okay; a little muscle soreness is common but joint pain is not.
- Dizziness and fainting may have several causes. These could be signs of low blood sugar. The best way to find out is to test the blood. If it is below 70, give food or fluid with sugar. If it isn't low, the symptoms could be signaling a need for fluids. If your buddy has been drinking sufficient water before and during exercise (see "Tips" later in this chapter for guidelines), it could be a heart or circulation problem. Get help.

Problems Are Rare

It's true that people with diabetes are at greater risk for heart attacks and that after reading the list of symptoms above, you may feel leery at the thought of exercising with someone with diabetes–thinking they may drop at your feet.

This is *not likely* to happen. It's even less likely, if your relative, friend or co-worker has been checked out by a physician before starting the exercise program and at the regular intervals his or her physician recommends.

Remember, lots of things can go wrong while you're driving, but you don't sit at home and miss all that's out there because there is a chance of an accident.

So here are the nuts and bolts of getting moving and learning to like it–together.

Types Of Exercise

Any moderate exercise (unless there is some health condition that makes it inadvisable) is better than no exercise. However, there are some kinds of exercise that are better than others. Aerobic exercise is exercise that uses oxygen. Aerobic exercise forces the heart and lungs to work hard enough to improve their strength but not so hard that they can't get enough oxygen and fuel to the tissues. It can be done for extended periods without becoming breathless.

Aerobic exercise is also continuous and rhythmical. Golfing and window-shopping aren't aerobic because they involve too much stopping. To strengthen the heart and lungs, they need to work at least 65% of their maximum capacity for a minimum of 20 minutes at a time.

An example of an intense anaerobic exercise is racing up a flight of stairs. You quickly get out of breath and exhausted because it demands more oxygen than your heart and lungs can supply. That kind of effort can't continue for more than a few minutes.

While most anaerobic exercise can strengthen muscles, increase flexibility, and be fun, it doesn't burn as many calories as aerobic exercise, nor does it have the best heart and lung strengthening effects.

Focusing on only one kind of exercise could get boring, so doing a variety is a good idea. Just give more time to aerobic activities. Here is a list of both types:

Aerobic	Anaerobic
Aerobic dancing	Archery
Bench stepping	Baseball
Bike riding	Basketball
Walking briskly	Bowling
Cross country skiing	Gardening
Jogging	Housework
Canoeing	Tennis
Swimming	Volleyball
Rowing	Weight lifting/
Rope skipping	resistance training

Even though some of the activities in the anaerobic column can be done at quite a strenuous level, there is usually a good bit of stopping and starting instead of the continuous, rhythmic movements in the aerobic column. Again, that doesn't mean they are useless, they just shouldn't be done to the exclusion of the activities in the first list.

Liking an activity is usually essential to keeping it up over time. No program will succeed if the person does not find the activity enjoyable and cannot become reasonably competent at it.

The characteristics of the individual have a bearing on whether it will be enjoyable and "doable." For example, for the obese and the elderly, swimming is easier on the joints than walking. Those with retinopathy (a diabetic eye complication) should avoid racquetball or tennis unless protective goggles are worn. Someone with poor circulation should avoid scuba diving because of the changes in atmospheric pressure.

That still leaves room for personal preference. The sky's the limit (though parachuting is not an aerobic activity) but keep in mind that expense and convenience can have an impact on how often the activity will be done. If the gym is too far away, or the facilities are too crowded, or the cost of ski lift tickets are too much of a financial strain, you and your buddy will find more excuses for *not* going than opportunities for going to the gym or the slopes.

Time For Exercise

One of the recommendations given to people who want to start and stay on an exercise program is to choose a time when it is convenient and apt to be done regularly. For people with diabetes, though, especially those who take diabetes medication, certain times of the day are better than others.

Exercise in the morning is more effective in increasing carbohydrate use from meals for the rest of the day. The best effects are felt the first 12 hours after exercise when the muscles are replenishing their energy stores by removing sugar from the blood.

For insulin and oral diabetes medication users, exercise in the later part of the day increases the risk of low blood sugar in the early morning hours while still asleep. That's why after a strenuous workout in the afternoon John eats a larger snack before he goes to bed.

However, for type 2 diabetics who are not on insulin or oral medication, after dinner exercise can be done without danger of having a low blood sugar at three in the morning. And it's an excellent way to use up the carbohydrate from that dinner (which tends to be a larger meal).

Intensity

When people start to exercise they often want to do a week's work in a day. But exercise at too intense a level means the lungs and heart can't keep up and in a few minutes the person is gasping, "I feel terrible, this can't be good for me."

It isn't. The heart is being strained to work at too high a level. And while a healthy heart can take the extra effort, the unpleasantness of the experience often turns off the exerciser.

There's a comfortable range of intensity that gets or keeps a person in shape without overdoing it and a couple of time-tested ways to judge if you and your buddy are working at an effective level.

The best known is by taking your pulse. For most people an effective exercise heart rate is between 65% and 80% of maximum heart rate.

Taking Your Own Pulse

To take your pulse, place the tips of your index and middle finger on the other hand where the thumb joins the hand. Slide the fingers past the hand and just onto the wrist. Let them rest with slight pressure side by side in the groove between the bone on the outside and the tendon on the wrist. Look at your watch and count the first beat as zero. Stop when 10 seconds have passed.

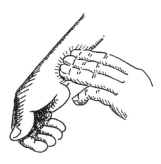

Another place to take your pulse is in your neck about one inch from the center of your throat. Again, use the index finger and the middle finger (don't use your thumb—it has a strong pulse of it's own and you might feel both beats).

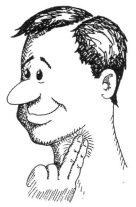

You'll be checking your pulse when you're exercising to determine if you're in your aerobic target range.

Calculating Your Aerobic Target Range

To calculate your effective effort level (target range), subtract your age from 220. That number is your maximum heart rate. You should not exercise at that rate–that's only for running away from tigers.

Once you have the maximum, multiply that number by 0.65 and again by 0.8. Those two numbers are the range your heart should beat in one minute while you're exercising. Here's the formula:

220 minus age = maximum heart rate
(in heart beats per minute)

Maximum heart rate x 0.65 = **lowest** effective
rate in heart beats per minute (65%)

Maximum heart rate x 0.80 = **highest** effective
rate in heart beats per minute (80%)

You really won't find beats per minute a very practical number to use, though. Who wants to count their pulse for a whole minute? Besides, if you stop what you're doing, your pulse slows down fairly quickly so by the end of the minute you won't be getting an accurate rate of what your pulse rate was while you were exercising. So most experts recommend taking your pulse for 10 seconds.

To calculate your range for a 10-second pulse, just divide six into the numbers you got for the 65% and 80% percent.

Example for someone 50 years old:

Maximum heart rate: $220 - 50 = 170$

$\boxed{\text{Minimum}}$ exercise heart rate per minute:
$170 \times 0.65 = 110$/beats/minute
Minimum exercise heart rate per 10 seconds:
Divide 110 by 6 = 18 beats/10 seconds

$\boxed{\text{Maximum}}$ exercise heart rate per minute:
$170 \times 0.8 = 136$ beats per minute
Maximum exercise heart rate per 10 seconds:
Divide 136 by 6 = 23 beats/10 seconds

From this calculation, the ideal range per 10 seconds is 18 to 23 beats per 10 seconds *for a 50 year old.* Remember to go through the calculations for your and your buddy's own ages.

Some Calculated Target Heart Rates at
65% and 80% of Maximum Heart Rate

Number of Heart Beats in 10
Seconds Level of Intensity

Age	65%	85%
20	22	27
25	21	26
30	21	25
35	20	25
40	20	24
45	19	23
50	18	23
55	18	22
60	17	21
65	17	21
70	16	21
75	16	19
80	15	19
85	15	18

This range (65 to 80% of maximum) may not be appropriate for everyone. Some may not be able to exceed 50%–especially not at first. Others who are very athletic, may aim for, and succeed at 90%. Your friend or family member with diabetes, and you too, should have a physician involved in the decision or how hard and how long to exercise.

Frequency and duration are factors in weight loss.

Exercise at 65-80% intensity level for at least 20 to 30 minutes will start burning fat instead of just the sugar stored in the muscles. If your diabetic friend or relative, or you, want to lose weight, exercise at least five days a week–six or seven *is* better.

You may have heard that every other day is enough exercise to stay healthy–and it is, to maintain cardiovascular strength. But not enough calories are burned to make much of a dent in body fat.

And recent research has shown that although 60 minutes per day may be enough to stabilize one's weight–to *lose* pounds, 90 minutes per day is necessary.

197

Even if weight loss is a goal, however, more is not better for everyone. The elderly recover more slowly from muscle exertion, so for them 45 minutes is usually a good maximum time. More than this can result in muscle aches.

If you don't like the aerobic target range method of determining if you're exercising at a useful intensity, see if you and your exercise buddy or buddies can talk comfortably and still walk. If you can, you're probably not exercising at too intense a level. Now, try to sing. If you can all sing, you're going too slowly. If you can talk but can't sing, that's perfect.

If your duet makes people throw money, don't stop.

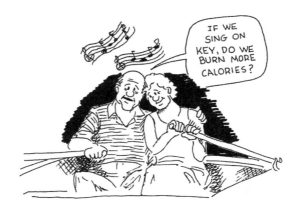

Weight training: good for all ages and sexes

Before you, or anyone with diabetes, start weight training get checked out by your health care provider. You may be pleasantly surprised to get an okay no matter what your age.

A recent Tufts University study was conducted with nursing home patients to learn if muscle strengthening through weight training could safely and effectively prevent falls due to weak muscles.

In just eight weeks those frail elders increased their muscle strength three to four times. As you might imagine, they were not mountain climbers: they had a myriad of health problems. Some had osteoarthritis (the kind of arthritis most common as we age), osteoporosis, high blood pressure, and heart disease. The oldest weight lifter was 101 years old.

When you hear the words, "weight lifter" does the image of a 400-pound, muscle-bulging man come to mind? It's not that kind of 200-pound barbell lifting that these senior citizens did.

They lifted hand weights, used stretchy bands, or moved their legs with weights strapped to their ankles.

Weight training together with aerobic exercise in a program is a very good combination. Aerobic activities are well recognized for their cardiovascular effects, cholesterol improvement, fat burning and other benefits. But muscle strengthening using weights is also a great help in maintaining physical fitness. It even helps with weight loss because more toned muscles mean more calories are burned, even at rest. More importantly, it helps prevent loss of calcium from bones, which can result in fractures and, as mentioned, fewer falls due to weak muscles.

Weight training requires at least a couple of soup cans (unopened) as hand weights to start. Extend and bend the arm slowly 10 times. If you feel as if you could easily do another 10 or 20, you need heavier weights.

But one pair of weights will probably not be enough. What your biceps can lift, your triceps won't budge. That's another reason why you brought your buddy. Between the two of you, you should be able to buy an adequate selection for every muscle group movement. Two different hand weights and one set of strap-on weights should get you started. Some sets are sold as handles with assorted weights that can be switched so you only have to buy one set of handles. Or there are strap-on weights for ankles or wrists that have little pockets for adding weights so many combinations are possible.

Generally, each exercise should be done slowly 10 times. Slow is better than fast because when you speed up, momentum takes away some of the effort. If you can do more than 12, add a bit more weight next time. It won't hurt you to do more than 12; it's just not an effective use of your exercise time. If 10 is too much, stop. You can rest or you can switch to a lighter weight, or do both. This is not like aerobics where continuous movement is necessary for maximum benefit. With weight training you can stop anywhere in the process.

You can learn what movements to make from a TV weight training show, or one of the many books or tapes in the library, video and book store. Or you can join a gym, or get a personal trainer. I know it sounds very Hollywoodish to have a personal trainer but they can be affordable, especially if you and your buddy or buddies split the fee. And you won't need a trainer every time you lift weights–just in the beginning when you're learning, and then once in a while as a refresher or when you want to try new equipment. A personal trainer will be able to tell you how to do each exercise correctly to prevent strains.

Weight training should never be done two days in a row. A day should pass between sessions to allow muscle cells to build new tissue. The nursing home weight lifters mentioned earlier, did their training three times a week with a day or two between.

If you are a woman, you may be dubious about weight training because you think you'll develop big, unfeminine muscles. That won't happen. You will tone your muscles but not make them noticeably larger. To do that you would have to lift huge barbells as Mr. America does. I guarantee that none of the nursing home ladies had their flannel nighties split from bulging arm muscles.

Exercise Machines

An exercise machine, like Pat's exercise bike, can be a real plus for an exercise program. Using one can work more parts of your body than your usual activity. For example, if you usually take walks, consider a rowing machine or ski exerciser that gives your upper body a challenge.

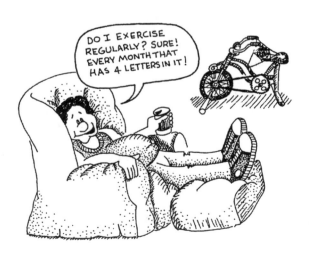

Another advantage of having a machine in your home is that it is always available. Pat likes hers because when it's raining or very hot she can pedal in comfort. I like my treadmill because I can read the paper, watch TV and do crossword puzzles, all while I burn lots of calories.

Try before you buy. There are a number of places where you can use the machines before you plunk down a bunch of money.

Community centers with exercise facilities are usually free and will give you some clues as to which machines you like.

Another place is a gym. Considering the price of some machines, it might be well worth a short membership in a gym just to be able to use their equipment and learn what works for you. They will also have an excellent selection: stair steppers, ski, rowing, and elliptical machines, in addition to the standard treadmills, etc. As a member, you'll also get some expert advice from their trainers to help you personalize your choice.

Stores will let you try out their equipment. Plan to use several machines briefly and a machine that you're serious about for at least 10 minutes at a low effort setting before you buy. If you know anyone who owns any of the machines you liked best, ask to use theirs for a longer period, two or three times.

There are companies which sell used fitness gear or rent machines. They are listed in the phone book and on-line under, "Fitness Equipment."

Whichever machine you decide on, it will require real effort in the beginning. It may almost seem like work (ugh). But it won't always be like that. When I first started using an exercise bike, it took a lot of grunting to do one mile. Even after a week or so, getting up to two and then three miles was almost as bad. But a wonderful thing happened when I could pedal five miles. It stopped being tough and started being automatic. I had evidently developed enough muscle strength in my thighs to make it comfortable.

The moral is *stick with it*; it won't always require the effort it does in the beginning.

Exercise Myths

There are some myths about exercise that are more than useless, as they can be downright harmful.

1. The first is that old favorite, **"No pain, no gain."** Exercise done correctly is not supposed to hurt joints. Some muscle soreness can be expected whenever you try some new activity but more than that is not desirable. It's not always possible to avoid overdoing it– sometimes we discover the next day that some move was a bit too much. It happens, but try not to make exercise unpleasant.

2. Another myth is that **if you don't exercise, your muscles will turn to fat.** Fat is fat and muscle is muscle, neither can become the other. What can happen, though, is that unexercised muscles will get a bit smaller and the normal fat layer will become thicker if excess calories are eaten.

3. Myth number three is that **the more you sweat, the better your exercise program is.** Sweat is water not fat. No matter how much you sweat, your body will only lose water. And that water will need to be replaced by drinking fluids to make up the loss. Rubber exercise suits that make you sweat more can be harmful. They defeat the purpose of sweating, which is to cool off the body by letting the sweat evaporate.

4. Another common myth is that **you can tell how well your exercise program is working by what your scale tells you.** Muscle weighs more than fat so you could lose five pounds of fat, feel your waistband get looser, and still not see any change in what the bathroom scale tells you. You lost fat and gained an equal weight in muscle but it will serve you much better. It will burn more calories while you're sleeping and muscle takes up less room so you will lose inches.

These myths and old wives tales can sabotage your and your buddy's exercise program. Believing them could make exercise so unpleasant you'd quit in a week, or so discouraging you'd quit in a month.

The expert on exercise and diabetes is an exercise physiologist. Your buddy's physician or the local affiliate of the American Diabetes Association should be able to recommend one. An exercise physiologist can evaluate the effect exercise has on your friend or family member's blood sugar and offer personalized advice.

Tips For Making an Exercise Program Work–Together

Imagine that your friend or relative has just left the doctor's office determined to have a better working body, get off the couch, and start an exercise program.

You know it's important for him or her to succeed, but you also know that turning from a couch potato into a lean, mean moving machine is a difficult transition which takes some time. How can you help? Here are some suggestions for maximizing the chances that exercise will become a life long habit.

1. **Do it together.** Together, exercise is a social event not just a chore, though it probably will seem like a chore in the beginning. The time when we as kids thought running and playing sports was fun gets replaced by the idea that exercise is a lot like work. Talking and sharing as a twosome or with others can put the pleasure back into moving our bodies. Even as kids we used to play tag and have races in neighborhood groups, didn't we?

Pat found that having her husband's company made all the difference. On the days when she didn't feel like walking, his "Let's go, it's a beautiful day," made her reluctant to disappoint him, so she went. On days he wasn't enthusiastic, she said, "Let's go, I like your company," and he went.

The main reason exercising with someone is better, is that it usually *is* more enjoyable, and having fun is the most important factor in keeping people exercising. Research studies have shown that while people *start* exercise programs for the health benefits, they *keep* exercising because of factors such as, friendship, encouragement, mental escape, competition and the surroundings.

It would not be a good idea for Pat's husband to suggest a walk saying it would help her blood sugar or waistline. Instead, he and you, would be better served by noticing and commenting that the exercise is pleasurable in itself. This includes not using the daily walk to discuss the family budget, gripes, or anything unpleasant. Use this time as a respite from everyday problems.

2. **Don't try to do too much too soon.** It's the one who is more out of shape that should set the pace. Pushing someone too fast will only make exercise an unpleasant experience and almost guarantee quitting.

Using the heart rate method can be helpful in the beginning. Covert Bailey in *The New Fit or Fat* tells the story of a 59-year old woman who said she tried to end a lifetime of taking it easy by running in place. She gave up after five days because every time she ran in place, she'd collapse after four minutes and feel terrible the rest of the day. She hadn't taken her pulse so she didn't know what intensity she'd been trying to work at.

Covert had her run in place for one minute–took her pulse for 10 seconds and found it was 28 instead of somewhere between 18 and 22, which would have been her safe, effective exercise range.

He had her try again just lifting her feet a few inches off the floor. This was still too much and she was soon panting.

Finally, he had her lift just her heels off the floor. That was perfect. It was the amount of effort that kept her in the target range without getting breathless.

This story illustrates how only a little movement in an unfit person can be the ideal starting place.

> **Whatever you do**
> **that's more than you used to do**
> **is going to make a difference**

3. **Choose a time that you both can regularly devote to exercise.** For co-workers, before or after work may be best. Lunchtime can be great. Take your lunch with you. Eat while you walk (take small bites, though).

Even though morning is best for insulin-dependent diabetics and after dinner is terrific for type 2 diabetics who don't take medication, if these times are not great for you and your buddy, do it when you can. Food and insulin can be changed to accommodate your exercise time, especially if it's regularly scheduled at that time and becomes routine.

4. **Get a pedometer (step counter).** It allows you to keep track of a day's movement without dedicating a fixed time to walking. Most Americans walk 3,000 to 3,500 steps a day. The recommended

goal is 10,000. If that seems daunting, start small and add just a bit each week. One study showed that just 2,000 steps more than you're doing now will take off about 10 pounds in a year.

First, though, you need an accurate pedometer. You can get a very good one for $15 to $25. More money means more features. If you just want to count steps and not miles or calculate calories, etc. you can get one closer to $15.

Clip the pedometer to a well-fitting waistband straight up from the knee. If your waistband is loose or you're wearing a dress, clip the pedometer onto your underpants. Pantyhose should go over the pedometer. Too much cushioning (clothes *or* body fat under the pedometer interferes with it's accurate counting so anyone with a protruding belly should clip it to the waistband at the small of the back. There's a little pendulum inside the device that won't work if it's resting on a "shelf."

For the first week assess the total number of steps taken during a normal day at home and/or work. Keep track at the end of the day and get the average at the end of the week.

The next week, add 500 or more steps a day. If you had to guess how long it would take you to walk 500 steps, what would you say? It's only five minutes for most of us.

The pedometer allows you to get credit for short walks such as five minutes of your break, walking in the hall, or around the building.

5. **Carry supplies.** Have fluids, food, a charged cell phone or change for a phone, and diabetic supplies (such as glucose tabs) with one or both of you and know what you should do in case your buddy has a low blood sugar.

Trained athletes make a point of drinking fluids regularly to replace the water lost through sweat and exhaling. Amateurs like us think if we're not thirsty, we don't need water. Not so. We can't depend on our sense of thirst to tell us when and how much to drink. This is especially true of older people whose sensation of thirst gradually becomes less reliable.

Here is the minimum amount of fluid you and your buddy will need when you're exercising. You will each need even more if it's hot or you're exercising strenuously:

> 1 cup of water 15 minutes before exercise
> ½ cup of water every 15 minutes of exercise
> 1 or more cups of water after exercise

An even more scientific method of learning how much water you need to replace is to weigh yourself before and after exercise. Drink two cups of water for every pound of weight loss.

6. Encourage your relative, friend or colleague to wear a medical I.D. bracelet (or buy one and give it to him or her). A diabetic emergency could happen when you are not there.

7. Set small goals, keep track of progress and give yourselves rewards for meeting those goals.
The goals could be minutes you spend exercising, blood sugar readings for your buddy, waist measurement, or blood pressure.

Goals need to be realistic and attainable. No measurement or weight goals of a 20 year old (unless you are a 20 year old) or perfect blood sugar level goals allowed. No four-minute miles, either. Goals like these would only make you and your buddy feel discouraged instead of uplifted.

Write down your starting numbers and add to your diary regularly. Don't zero in on the occasional sags in progress. However, if regular barriers, e.g. rainy days, prevent your walks, some problem solving may be necessary. Here in the rainy part of Oregon we have a saying, "There is no such thing as a day that's too wet. You just need better rain gear." But if you don't like that idea, walking in the mall can substitute.

Take a good look at what the general trend is toward your goals—don't get too hung up on the occasional misses. And realize that plateaus happen.

Decide on rewards for attaining your goals and the give them to yourself. I bet the first reward you thought of was food. We do seem to think that way. Cookies are common rewards kids get for good behavior. You don't have to eliminate food as a reward, though. A cup of non-fat, sugar-free frozen yogurt wouldn't be *bad,* but try to think up a reward that you could both enjoy that *doesn't* involve food. Do any of these sound good to you?

1. Massages
2. Book on tape or favorite music CD
3. A weekend at a favorite resort
4. A new exercise outfit
5. Tickets to a concert
6. _____

8. Start your own exercise library. Buy or borrow exercise CDs, or record exercise programs from your own TV for home exercise and weight training. Buying a professional exercise video has one big drawback. After you and your buddy have heard the same advice, or worse, the cute comment of the host over and over, it will sound like fingernails on a blackboard. You can borrow CDs from a video store and even the library, and you probably should before buying one anyway. They come in all levels of difficulty for different ages and physical abilities.

And if you're alternating an aerobics show with a weight training show, you get even more variety.

Consider swapping CDs with other exercisers. You'll learn from each other what features are most important, like level of intensity, music, sitting exercises, interesting patter, sexy outfits and so forth.

9. Wii computer fitness, sports and dance. Wii allows you to have a multitude of sports (bowling, tennis, slalom skiing, and many more), dances, and fitness programs and assessments in your home in front of a TV. This new technology can be very useful and is not just for kids who like to bounce around. Retirement homes and extended care facilities use them to broaden the exercise choices for their residents.

It's a great new excuse to get together with friends and compete with heart healthy benefits you don't get from canasta or charades.

Another plus is impressing the kids in your life. One 12-year old said, "Let's visit grandpa, he plays video games."

10. Be open to suggestions from each other on new ways to exercise. Variety is a key to keeping exercise interesting. Doing different activities also means different muscle groups get challenged and over-all fitness is greater than if you only do one thing all the time. This is called cross training.

Several years ago my husband wistfully mentioned that he'd like to have a canoe or a rowboat. I wasn't very encouraging. The idea of paddling around in a boat did nothing for me. I didn't mind if he got one but I wasn't going to join him.

He still doesn't have his boat, or look at ads regularly, or even mention it anymore.

How different this scenario would have been if, when he mentioned his boating wish, I had said, "Let's get one, it might be fun." He would have felt less constrained about spending the money and time to get a boat because it would have been for *us*. And who knows, I might have loved paddling a canoe or rowing. Together, it would have been more than just exercise.

11. Wet, cold or hot weather doesn't mean you have to give up your walk with your buddy.

If there's an enclosed mall near you, it is a great rainy, snowy, or hot weather option. It also is a good choice for someone who needs an even surface underfoot.

Do one brisk lap of a floor without stopping and note how long that takes. If it takes 10 minutes and your usual walk is one hour, do five more laps. This timing allows you to stop, if you need a bathroom or other essential break, without getting into an argument about how much time you still need to walk. Notice I said, "essential" break. If you're trying to keep your heart rate up for a true aerobic workout, you can't stop frequently.

The time to stop and browse is when you've finished your laps. That's one of the advantages of mall walking. It provides a built-in reward for your good work. You can shop, browse, and people watch all you want *after* you've reached your goal.

Final Bits Of Advice

Three ways to start your own exercise program:
1. Buy a pedometer
2. Join a square dancing group
3. Borrow a two year old

Three ways to increase your buddy's exercise level:
1. Start walking together in a mall three times a week
2. Join a swimming club with a two for the price of one offer
3. Buy her a puppy right after she gets new carpeting

13

Sex, Love, and Diabetes:
Not Just Hormones

Picture this scene. Two honeymooners are in bed cuddling after making love. Before dropping off to sleep, the bride, Brooke, says, "If I get shaky and sweaty in the middle of the night, feed me some of the candy I put in the night stand drawer." His reply: "No, I won't do that, I know you have diabetes and you're not allowed to eat candy."

Why would Brooke think she might get sweaty and shaky; why tell him to give her candy; and why would he refuse?

Sex Is Exercise

Passionate sex can require a good deal of physical activity and that means muscles are at work. For muscles to do "work," they need glucose (sugar) for fuel. The first place muscles get sugar is from what's stored inside muscle cells. After that's gone, they take it up from the blood stream. Any significant, sustained physical activity means more sugar going to muscles and less circulating in the blood. And since sex can be pretty physically demanding, there's a good chance it will lower blood sugar.

The tricky part is trying to predict if it will get too low, avoiding the low, or recognizing it early and dealing with it. The shakiness and sweatiness the bride told her hubby to look out for, are symptoms of low blood sugar. They are "signals" caused by the release of adrenalin (an alarm hormone) and the adrenalin's message is, "Something is not O.K. Fix it."

Recognizing and Correcting Low Blood Sugar

Shakiness and sweatiness are two of the more obvious signs that blood sugar is getting too low. Some signs can only be felt by the person with diabetes, while others are detectable by a partner who knows what to look for. Here are symptoms that can be seen by a partner:

shakiness	clumsiness
sweatiness	confusion
complaints of hunger	seizure
behavior changes	loss of consciousness

Usually a person with diabetes can feel when he or she is "getting low" and take steps to check and correct it. But, as you can see from the list above, some of the symptoms, such as confusion, may make it impossible for the person with a low blood sugar to do anything about it. This is a time when an informed partner can help.

Fortunately, one of the earliest visible symptoms is sweating–a very useful signal of low blood sugar. Sweating cools the body so what often happens in bed, is that the one feeling cold will look for warmth by snuggling close to the warmer body. Hopefully, this will wake the "snugglee" and clue him or her to the need to do something to raise their partner's blood sugar.

That's where the candy or other form of sugar in the night stand drawer comes in. Sugar in this instance is actually medicine. Here are some of the foods that many folks keep around to raise their blood sugar (the generally recommended amounts to give are in parenthesis):

LifeSavers (6 to7 or about half a roll)
glucose tablets (3 or 4 or whatever number totals 15 grams carbohydrate)
glucose gel (whatever amount will give 15 grams carbohydrate)
¼ to ⅓ cup raisins
½ cup fruit juice or *regular* soda (*not* sugar-free)

Ideally, it's best to test blood sugar. If it's less than 60 or 70[1], give 15 grams of carbohydrate and wait 15 minutes. If the person is not feeling better by then, or if blood sugar is still not over 70, give another 15 grams and wait another 15 minutes.

But if you don't have a meter handy, or don't know how to use one, give 15 grams of carbohydrate anyway.

There is no point in giving a larger amount–it won't make the blood sugar normalize more quickly and it might well make it go too high later. Sometimes it takes 30 to 45 minutes for the person with the low blood sugar to feel O.K. again–even though their blood sugar has returned to normal. Because of this delay in feeling right again, the best way to judge if someone is out of danger is to do a blood glucose test. Knowing how to test can come in very handy. Ask your partner to show you how to test him or her and ask if you may do a test from time to time to keep in practice.

If you should happen to find the person unconscious, do not try to pour fluids down his or her throat or give food. It is very dangerous to give anything by mouth to anyone who can't naturally swallow.

Some people think it's OK to rub some glucose gel or honey on the inside of the mouth of an unconscious person or one having a seizure. But, not everyone agrees that a significant amount of sugar gets into the blood stream this way. Worse, most of the glucose gel will "melt" and go down the esophagus. On the way down, it can be aspirated (breathed) into the lungs–a potentially very serious medical problem. Even the manufacturers of glucose gel warn against using it on an unconscious person or anyone having a seizure.

Instead of risking food or fluid "going down the wrong way" in someone who is unconscious or having a seizure, call for emergency help, *immediately* get him or her to an emergency room, or, if you know how, give an injection of glucagon. (See Chapter 9 for more on low blood sugar).

---

[1] Some sources say treat a low at 60, others say 70.

Anticipating Low Blood Sugar

Lest you think that sex automatically leads to emergencies, it doesn't. It's even less likely once folks with diabetes learn what to do to prevent their blood sugar from getting too low.

Daria says, "As far as sex goes, I had to learn the hard way that it's a form of exercise. My doctor didn't warn me that during or after having sex I could have low blood sugar. Now I keep a candy dish by my bed or if I know it's about to get hot and heavy I excuse myself and go to the kitchen and drink a half cup of orange juice and I'm ready to go."

Barbara says that when she and her husband give each other that "special look," she tests her blood. If it's on the low side, she says, "Sorry, I have to eat something first." He understands by now that her snack is good insurance against having their pleasure interrupted to treat low blood sugar.

Jeanette is also a big believer in prevention. Her short and sweet advice is, "Eat first, play around later."

Food isn't just for before, either. "Food can be part of the hot and heavy," advises Kerrie, but just in case I do get low, I always keep a pack of LifeSavers by the bed or Cliff will get me something if it's sudden and severe."

Preventing low blood sugar isn't just to avoid the nuisance and possible danger. After many years with diabetes, Cyndee says, "I check my blood sugar while I'm washing up before sex, to make sure it's above 80 or I will not be able to have an orgasm."

By the way, the bride Brooke is no longer married to the groom who wouldn't give her candy–for that, and some other reasons.

Embarrassment

Barbara, Jeanette, and Kerrie are in long-term relationships; to them low blood sugar is a nuisance, not an embarrassment.

However, it can be embarrassing for folks who are with new partners they haven't yet educated about their diabetes.

William remembers an occasion when he was madly kissing a girl in his apartment. He was looking forward to taking her to bed when he started feeling himself getting low. Because he was too embarrassed to tell her what was really happening, he stopped kissing her and mumbled something about not feeling well. She left perplexed and somewhat miffed, and he got the glass of juice. After that night, he matter-of-factly told his dates the truth–it was better than missing out on their company.

What is the source of William's and many other folks' embarrassment? Ava can help us understand.

Ava says she feels she's imposing when she has to interrupt sex because of her blood sugar. It's not something a person without diabetes has to deal with and she hates being unique–especially during intimate moments. She remembers one time in particular. She and her new partner were having a lovely time in bed when she felt symptoms of low blood sugar. She had to stop the action, run downstairs, get orange juice, and wait a ½ hour before they could get back to "business." Her low blood sugar didn't ruin the evening, but the prolonged reassurances she needed from her lover about her "problem" almost did.

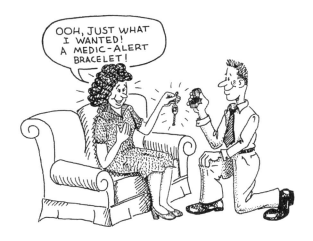

When Valerie revived her relationship with her old boyfriend she neglected to tell him how her newly-diagnosed diabetes might affect them. The first weekend they spent together, she didn't eat enough. "I felt weak, dizzy, and shaky most of the day, so I didn't feel much like getting out of bed. He took that as a sign that he "wore me out." I never actually told him what the real problem was."

Rapturous feelings and embarrassment or not, diabetes can't be ignored.

Alcohol and Low Blood Sugar

One of the more common contributing factors to low blood sugar is alcohol. Low blood sugar can happen during sex, not only because of the exercise involved but also because drinking alcohol is often part of the ritual of having sex.

Alcohol contributes to low blood sugar because when we drink alcohol, the liver stops doing one of its most important jobs, which is to release stored sugar when it's needed. This is not a problem for people who don't take insulin or other medications that lower blood sugar, their pancreases just stop putting out insulin when their blood sugar gets low. Normally, if our blood sugar gets too low (for example, whenever we go several hours without food) our liver supplies us with sugar to tide us over until we eat.

But combine blood-sugar-lowering medications with a liver that's busy processing alcohol–and you get blood sugar than can get very low. The more alcohol, the longer the effect, so it's not unheard of for people to get a seriously low blood sugar several hours after drinking, when whatever food they ate earlier has been absorbed and there's very little glucose left in the blood stream. Adding the exercise of love-making makes a low even more likely.

Another problem with alcohol is that many people drink to feel mellow or tipsy, in short, to feel carefree. But feeling free of their cares means they are less likely to attend to the various decisions that are necessary to keep their blood sugar in control. Who, after two or three drinks, is likely to think about testing their blood sugar, to snack if it's on the low side, to tell their partner what the symptoms of low blood sugar are and what to do if he or she gets them?

Want to give your partner a drink that will help prevent low blood sugar during love-making? Give him or her a glass of fruit juice or milk. Both have carbohydrate to provide glucose.

Or peel your honey 15, or so, grapes. Just kidding. You don't have to peel the grapes but wouldn't that earn you lots of "points"?

High Blood Sugar

If sex usually lowers blood sugar, can it be used as a treatment for high blood sugar?

Cyndee says for her it can–and does. "Sex *always* lowers my blood sugar, so if it's elevated and I want to tease my husband, I tell him that I need sex to bring my blood sugar down. This allows him to feel that there are some ways he can be of help to me."

Although Cyndee almost makes diabetes sound like a sexual turn-on, the reality, especially for newcomers to diabetes like Theresa and Art can be very different.

For weeks before their September wedding Art was thirsty, urinated a lot, was sluggish, and didn't feel well. He didn't do anything about it though. Both he and Theresa thought that getting away on their honeymoon would fix everything. It didn't turn out that way though. On their wedding night and every night in their honeymoon suite, Theresa put on a sexy negligee and every night Art ignored her or said something like, "Aren't you cold in that thing?"

Theresa felt devastated. Before their wedding, they'd had a healthy sex life. But in the three months after they got married, they only made love twice. What caused Art's disinterest? High blood sugar from his undiagnosed diabetes. When he was finally diagnosed after Christmas and Theresa mentioned their practically non-existent sex life to the doctor, his brief answer was, "It's the diabetes. Be patient, things will improve."

And they did. Two days of insulin and Art was his old self.

But whenever Art's diabetes got out of control, their sex life went out the window. If his blood sugar was very high, he'd again feel so tired that even sex was too much of an effort. And when his blood sugar was too low, he wouldn't be able to get an erection.

Art's tiredness whenever his blood sugar was high is common. When a shortage of insulin results in the sugar staying in the blood instead of fueling the body's cells, they don't work well.

Keeping blood sugar in the normal range can pay off in more energy.

Birth Control

Bringing a child into the world with a devastating birth defect such as spina bifida or a severe heart defect is every parent's worse nightmare. For the huge majority of parents, this is not something they could have predicted–it happens to two to three of every 100 babies of mothers who don't have diabetes.

For women with diabetes, however, if a baby is conceived and develops while the mother's blood sugar is above normal during the first 6 weeks of pregnancy, the chances that the baby will have a major birth defect are significantly higher. Studies show the odds as low as 4 in 100 and as high as 22 out of 100. Generally, the higher the mother's average blood sugar, the greater the incidence of serious birth defects. So, almost all of those unhappy outcomes were preventable. The key is that **no woman with diabetes should have an unplanned pregnancy**. Conscientious use of a reliable birth control method **every single time** a woman has sexual intercourse is an absolute must.

Women who are contemplating pregnancy are urged to get their diabetes in excellent control *before* stopping their birth control. It's a lot of work but it's the best chance their baby has of avoiding serious birth defects. (Please see the Chapter 14 on pregnancy for details.)

There is no birth control method currently on the market that is generally contraindicated for women with diabetes. Years ago, oral contraceptives were not recommended because when they were first launched, "the pill" contained high dosages of estrogen and progestin, either of which when taken in large amounts can raise blood sugar. Recent studies show that newer low-dose birth control pills have almost no impact on blood sugar but may still be risky if a woman smokes or has cardiovascular, eye, or kidney complications. To use or not to use them is a decision she and her doctor should make after weighing her particular situation and history.

Individual considerations aside, the major downside to the safer low-dose pills is that missing a single pill, especially in midcycle, can result in pregnancy. To be protected in case of a missed pill, the woman should use another contraceptive method for the rest of the cycle and call the doctor to find out how to restart the pill.

Many women are not aware that a lot of medicines (Actos and Avandia for diabetes, antibiotics, sleeping pills, and antiseizure drugs, to name just a few), and anything that interferes with the pills absorption from the digestive tract, such as diarrhea or a dose of mineral oil, can result in a surprise pregnancy. How can you or your partner know if a particular medicine can decrease a contraceptive's strength or have some other drug interaction? Either of you can ask a pharmacist. And when in any doubt about the pills's dependability—use an additional contraceptive (such as condoms with contraceptive jelly) for the rest of the cycle.

There are other birth control options—some more reliable than others. Combining two methods (such as using a condom or diaphragm along with a spermicidal jelly) significantly increase the efficacy of any one method used alone.

New FDA-approved options include monthly hormonal injections, a vaginal hormone ring, or a weekly skin patch that delivers hormones.

When considering a contraceptive method, reliability, safety, convenience, and cost are all considerations that deserve to be discussed—with your partner and his or her physician.

If cost is an issue, be sure the doctor knows. Birth control varies significantly from one time costs (about $750 for a vasectomy) to $2,000 for 5 years of pills, patches, etc.

Lack of Desire and Depression

Remember Art's disinterest in sex on his honeymoon? Well, it's not just men who are affected by lack of desire when their blood sugar is too high, too low, or are not feeling their best for physical or emotional reasons.

Serena says, "I have problems with my blood sugar going way up and way down. Over and over. It affects my love life. Sometimes I don't want sex at all." Further complicating her love life is her unhappiness with her weight. She's not sure if she's depressed because she's overweight or is overweight because she's depressed.

Either is possible. Hearing the words, "You have diabetes" is sometimes all it takes to bring on sadness. Having *any* chronic disease can be depressing—and diabetes with it's restrictions and extra burdens can bring with it a sense of loss and occasionally helplessness. Depression can make sticking to a meal plan or exercise program seem impossible.

Additionally, diabetes causes chemical changes that make a person more likely to suffer from clinical depression.

Symptoms of depression include increased appetite (or lack of appetite), sleeping too much (or too little), chronic fatigue, trouble concentrating, poor memory, and loss of interest and enjoyment in social activities that once were enjoyable.

Ruby didn't think she was depressed until she read a list of the symptoms in her doctor's examining room. When the doctor came into the room she said, "I have practically every symptom on that list." The doctor prescribed an anti-depressant but warned her that the pills would probably make her feel worse before they made her feel better.

Ruby said that after about 3½ weeks the change was amazing. "I felt like a new person with energy I hadn't had in years. The best part was how it improved my marriage. I used to be terribly irritable with my husband. Not being depressed changed how I felt about him and lots of other things."

If depression could be the cause of extreme fatigue and other troubling symptoms, it deserves a doctor's attention. And it doesn't have to involve long, expensive psychotherapy. Brief, symptom-focused counseling with or without antidepressant drugs are both effective treatments and are frequently covered by insurance.

If the tiredness is due to high blood sugar, good diabetes care and patient education are indicated and will help physically and mentally. Any or all of the following could help: more frequent blood sugar monitoring, an adjustment of diabetes medication, a review of the diet, an exercise program, and perhaps stress management or psychological support.

Complications that Cause Sexual Problems

Sexual dysfunction can also be caused by nerve and circulatory damage. Some men can have problems getting and keeping erections, while some women with diabetes can have problems affecting desire, arousal, and orgasm, or pain with sexual intercourse.

Men: Erection Problems

Getting and keeping an erection and ejaculating normally depends on the penis getting a good blood supply and having properly functioning nerves. Both circulation and nerves can be damaged by diabetes, smoking, and alcoholic beverages. Some diabetic men find it impossible to get an erection. Others are able to get an erection but have problems maintaining it or ejaculating.

Fortunately, there are ways to remedy or at least slow down the causes of diabetes-related impotence. The first four priorities are to get blood sugar and blood fat (cholesterol, etc.) levels as close to normal as possible, stop smoking, and stop, or cut down on, alcoholic beverages.

Another culprit may be medication for hypertension, since blood pressure-lowering drugs can affect erections. Though it's dangerous to stop taking them if they're needed, switching to another or a combination of the newer hypertension drugs may control a man's blood pressure without affecting his erections. Other drugs can also cause impotence, especially tranquilizers and antidepressants.

Psychological factors such as depression, job stress, financial problems, and marital conflict used to be thought to cause most impotence. Psychological factors are actually to blame only about 10% of the time. The physician working together with a sex therapist can develop an evaluation and treatment plan. Blood and other tests may help determine if the cause is physical or psychological. With counseling and a supportive partner, erectile problems can sometimes be completely reversible.

Hormone deficiency is found in only about 3% of cases of impotence. A blood test can confirm or rule out the possibility. Sometimes it can be cured with testosterone patches or injections. However, before receiving testosterone replacement, and periodically while being treated, men should be carefully screened for prostate cancer with blood tests and rectal exams.

Other treatments and aids for impotence include oral medication, hand vacuum pumps, penile injections, urethral suppositories and surgical implants.

Injections of alprostadin into the side of the penis (scary-sounding but usually painless) are effective and relatively inexpensive. After an initial injection in the doctor's office to determine the proper dose; the man (or his partner) can learn to do the injections. Although injection treatment is usually safe, bruising and scar formation caused by the needle may occur and require ending the treatment. Also, in the remote case of the man's erection lasting more than 4 hours, he'd need a urologist's attention.

Alprostadil, the same drug that's used in penile injections can also be given as a suppository through a hollow plastic applicator inserted about one inch into the penis. The suppositories are less effective than the injections and more expensive, but are less intimidating than sticking a needle into one's penis.

Don's experience points out how many times, more than one option may need to be tried. "My doctor tested my hormone levels and since they were a bit low, he prescribed testosterone injections. They didn't help. I tried that vacuum pump next and although it allowed my wife and me to have intercourse, it seemed too mechanical." (The pump involves the use of an external vacuum device and one or more rubber tension bands. The vacuum chamber is placed over the unerect penis, and a pump or a hand bulb is used to evacuate air from the vacuum chamber, producing an erection. Once an adequate erection is produced, a kind of rubber band is slipped around the base of the penis to restrict the outflow of blood from the penis, thus maintaining the erection.)

Hoping to have a more "natural" experience, Don said he had high hopes that the impotence pill Viagra would work. Unfortunately, Don fell into the 30 to 50% of men for whom it doesn't work; even the maximum dosage didn't produce enough stiffness for intercourse.

Even when the impotence pill works, and even when side effects such as dangerous drops in blood pressure are not a concern, it has a major drawback–it's quite expensive–around $10 for the usual dose. In fact, all the treatments are at least somewhat costly. The penile suppository runs about $20 per use, the vacuum pump one-time cost is $300 to $400 (from a medical supplies source, less from a sex paraphernalia outlet), and surgery for penile implants costs $10,000 and up. When a man's insurance plan doesn't pay for the treatment, "cheap fun" can become an expensive proposition.

Reimbursement for impotence treatments varies among insurance carriers. Some pay for injections but not for suppositories. Others pay for the $10 pill but only a few per month.

Money aside, before choosing a method, it's always a good idea to discuss the options with one's partner. What might seem a dandy idea to one person, may not be acceptable to the other. For example, the vacuum device that Don found too "unnatural" is used by thousands of men with success. It has almost no medical downside (provided the rubber band is not left on for more than 30 minutes), is relatively inexpensive, and can be very effective. With the exception of the impotence pill, all the available methods take some getting used to–so don't give up too soon unless you or your partner feels very negatively about a particular method.

Don and his wife eventually opted for a penile implant. The surgery appears to generally provide safe and satisfying results. Before the operation, Don underwent a thorough check-up to rule-out likely causes of surgical complications plus he made sure his blood sugar was in excellent control so he would heal well.

Don's satisfaction with the procedure a year later? "It was worth every penny and even the mild temporary discomfort. Our loving is better than ever."

One of the saddest outcomes of impotence is how it frequently distances men from their partners.

Paulo was so humiliated when for the third time in a month he couldn't get an erection, that from then on, whenever his wife

Angela made him a special dinner or cuddled up to him (possible signs that she might be in the mood to make love) he'd pick a fight.

She interpreted his distance and rejection as her fault, or that Paulo was having an affair, never suspecting their deteriorating relationship was a result of his diabetes.

Paulo finally got the courage to ask his doctor for help—4 years later!

Communicating his feelings earlier to his wife and his physician would have saved a great deal of unhappiness.

He eventually found an acceptable treatment, but if he hadn't he could still have had an intimate relationship with his wife in ways that don't require an erection. Many men don't know that it's possible to have an orgasm without an erection. Or that caressing and kissing can satisfy one's need for closeness without intercourse.

Women's Sexual Complications

Bladder and Vaginal Infections

Women with diabetes that's not in good control, are more likely to have bladder and vaginal infections than nondiabetic women because high sugar levels provide more food for bacteria, fungi, and parasites. Both conditions can impact sexual pleasure and even affect a woman's general health.

Elizabeth says she went through a period when she had yeast or bladder infections every month for over a year. And, if that wasn't bad enough, the infections made her blood sugar high. "When my sugar is high, I'm irritable, bitchy, mean, and tired. I get overwhelmed with the smallest of details or responsibilities. And forget any relations with my husband."

The symptoms of a bladder infection are frequent, urgent, and painful urination, sometimes with blood-tinged urine. The first line of treatment is usually a sulfa drug. That usually brings significant relief within 4 hours of the first dose. One caution is that sulfa is from the same drug family as the sulfonylureas that many people with type 2 diabetes take to lower their blood sugar. The two drugs together can increase the effect of the sulfonylurea. Urge your partner to check with her physician or pharmacist and be prepared to check her blood sugar more often.

Some simple measures can help prevent bladder infections:

1. Keeping blood sugar in good control,
2. Washing hands and genitals of both participants before sex,
3. Emptying the bladder before and after sex,
4. Drinking lots of fluids.

Vaginal infections are usually, but not always, caused by yeast. When a yeast fungus is the culprit, the woman usually sees a white, cheesy vaginal discharge with a peculiar yeasty odor (similar to bread dough). She may have severe itchiness, burning, redness, swelling of the vaginal area, and painful sexual intercourse.

The same yeast organism that can infect the vagina can also grow in other warm, moist areas including under the breasts or in the creases between the legs and abdomen, the insides of the thighs and around the anus.

Because at least half a dozen organisms (including chlamydia and trichomonas), can infect the vagina and cause confusingly similar symptoms, a woman shouldn't rush to use an over the counter product that only treats yeast. Instead, she should be examined by her physician who can properly collect a sample of the secretion and examine it under a microscope.

A woman's partner must also be tested and treated, otherwise he can reinfect her.

In addition to taking the appropriate medication to kill the specific organism that is causing the infection, keeping the affected skin dry and blood sugar in good control will speed healing.

Vaginal infections are *more likely* to occur with birth control pill use, after antibiotic and cortisone medications, and with frequent vaginal douching; and *less likely* with daily bathing, wiping correctly from front to back after using the toilet, and wearing cotton panties.

Vaginal Dryness

Vaginal dryness is a common problem for women especially after menopause when estrogen levels decrease markedly. In women with diabetes who are still menstruating, dryness may be due to nerve damage which inhibits lubrication. Decreased libido (from disrupted hormone levels during poor diabetes control) can also contribute to dryness because sexual excitement is the stimulus for natural vaginal lubrication. Though it doesn't sound like a big deal, a dry vagina can cause severe discomfort during intercourse.

The easiest fix is to apply an over the counter vaginal lubricant before intercourse. Cyndee has a very creative method. "Since I'm usually quite dry even if I'm very stimulated, my husband and I have made a game out of applying lubricant. I have him use his penis like a paint brush and paint me with it. This way the application is like a game and stimulates both of us!"

Heidi has not had good results from ordinary lubricant. "I'm a very dry person from head to toe and even when I apply outside lubrication it dries up quickly within my vagina."

But a water-based vaginal lubricant such as K-Y Jelly is not the only option. For severe dryness, a vaginal suppository such as Lubrin can be inserted before foreplay. Replens is a newer product which provides 2 to 3 days relief from vaginal dryness with each application. It has an added bonus of maintaining a favorable vaginal pH–a help in decreasing recurrent yeast infections.

After menopause vaginal elasticity and lubrication can improve significantly with estrogen replacement, though its long-term use in pills with progesterone is no longer recommended because it increases risk of certain cancers. Lower dosages of estrogen are available in the form of patches, vaginal rings or cream.

Finding Help for Sexual Problems

Embarrassment is the number one barrier to getting help. If the problem is high or low blood sugar, the expert to consult is a physician who is interested in diabetes. If a specialist is needed, ask for a referral to an endocrinologist. They are frequently assisted by nurse practitioners or diabetes educators who can help stabilize blood sugar levels and other aspects of diabetes management.

For impotence, the initial testing and treatment can be tackled by the physician who gives general care. The next step is to consult a urologist.

For depression, the primary care provider is, again, the first person to consult. He or she can spell out the pros and cons of various choices in treatment (medication, counseling, etc.).

A gynecologist can help women with physical problems and referrals for depression.

In short, it's communication with one's partner and health care providers that can lead to a solution.

14

Pregnancy: A Labor of Love

Pregnancy and Type 1 Diabetes

For most women who have babies, taking care of their pregnancy starts when they know they're pregnant. Not so for 23 year old Shauna who has had type 1 diabetes for seven years. Giving herself and her baby the best care possible started months before she got pregnant.

Her endocrinologist (diabetes specialist) told her that it was especially important to keep her blood sugar normal when the fetus is conceived and for the critical 12 weeks afterward when its organs are being formed. This is the period when high blood sugars can cause serious birth defects, especially of the heart, nervous system and bones.

During the rest of the pregnancy, Shauna was careful to keep her blood sugar near normal to prevent the fetus from growing too large for her uterus to support. An overly large baby could have led to a premature labor. Many babies born to mothers with diabetes are large, fat babies. That's because they start producing their own insulin at about the 26th week of pregnancy and will process the extra sugar that they receive through the placenta from mom. That excess sugar will be stored as fat so they grow big and fat. Unfortunately, they are not as ready to be born as their sizes would suggest.

Fat babies mean more difficult labors and births with all the problems these entail for both the mothers and the babies.

Shauna's baby girl was full-term and weighed 7½ pounds. This may not seem like a weight to brag about, but when babies are born to mothers with diabetes, a normal birth weight is excellent. We know from the baby's weight that Shauna did a good job of keeping her blood sugar in a normal range, otherwise the baby might have weighed nine or ten pounds or more, and might have had problems.

Very big babies born prematurely due to their large weight may have breathing difficulties because of their immature lungs. Further, before birth they grow used to lots of sugar from the mother with her high blood sugar and produce an oversupply of insulin to handle that sugar. Then, after they are born and the mothers' sugar is cut off, their extra insulin makes their own blood sugar drop too low. If the medical team expects this low blood sugar, it can be planned for and the baby can be kept in the hospital for observation and weaning from its dependence on lots of sugar. In a matter of a couple of days, its insulin production will be normal. Without this planning, for example, if the mom had no prenatal care, the baby could suffer seizures, mental retardation, etc.

During pregnancy an expectant mother with diabetes is more likely to get ketoacidosis (See Chapter 10 on high blood sugar), a kidney infection, or preeclampsia (a complication of pregnancy that causes high blood pressure and seizures). Any of these could require hospitalization. Pregnancy can also contribute to a worsening of kidney and eye diseases. Advanced coronary artery disease is also associated with a higher death rate in pregnant women with diabetes. These are all risks that can be evaluated and discussed by the future mom and her physician.

Shauna didn't have any of these complications because she was healthy and she and her doctors were very careful. She checked her blood sugar often (5 to 10 times a day is not an unusual recommendation), visited her obstetrician every two weeks for the first eight months and then weekly. She had five or six ultrasound tests, weekly tests of the fetus's heart rate after the 28th week, an A1c blood test monthly, an eye test, and three urine tests that required she collect all her urine for 24 hours. After the 28th week she also counted the fetus's movements for 30 to 60 minutes and recorded the time of day at which she felt 10 fetal movements. If there had been any decrease in the fetus's activity, she would have called her doctor.

Shauna and most women with diabetes who want a baby, work hard to give it the best possible start. Ideally, they also have an experienced health-care team to help. The team should include a diabetes specialist, an obstetrician, a pediatrician or neonatologist, a diabetes educator nurse, and a dietitian.

Doctors who don't know how far pregnancy care for diabetes has come in the last 20 years, still believe and say, "You should adopt; women with diabetes can't have babies." The first obstetrician Shauna saw when she was considering getting pregnant said those very words to her. Now when Shauna plays with four-year-old Kristen, who is healthy and happy, she's glad she looked for a doctor with the most current information.

Type 2 Diabetes

Women with type 2 diabetes need to follow almost all the recommendations that apply to those with type 1. That is, they need to plan their pregnancies so that conception occurs when their blood sugar is within the normal range, they need to continue to keep their blood sugar within the guidelines, and they need to be monitored frequently to catch problems that could put their or the fetus' health at risk. They may even have to test for ketones.

What may come as an unpleasant surprise is that oral diabetes medications, with the possible exception of metformin, are stopped before conception and insulin started.

Gestational Diabetes

Shauna had type 1 diabetes long before she had her baby. But there is a kind of diabetes that comes during pregnancy and almost always goes away when the pregnancy is over. It's gestational diabetes.

It happens because the hormones produced by the placenta during pregnancy cause resistance to insulin. In 3 to 10% of pregnant women, their pancreases cannot produce enough extra insulin to meet the additional demand, so their blood sugars go up. Since they produce some insulin, they frequently don't have the symptoms of high blood sugar (thirst, weight loss, etc.) that typically signal type 1 diabetes. Their diabetes is more silent, and can go unnoticed if not looked for. In the past, doctors would be alert to a woman's risk if she had already had a baby weighing more than nine pounds. Nowadays, physicians don't stand by helplessly waiting for the birth of an overly large baby, with all the risks that entails. Between the 24th and 28th week of pregnancy they routinely test by having a woman drink 50 grams of glucose, wait an hour and then test her blood sugar. A woman who doesn't have gestational diabetes would be able to process that sugar without her blood sugar going up.

Women most at risk for gestational diabetes are obese, over 30 years of age, Hispanic, African American, or Native American, have a family history of diabetes, have prediabetes, or have already given birth to a baby over nine pounds.

Fortunately, gestational diabetes develops only in the later stage of pregnancy so at conception and the first three months, blood sugar is not elevated. Birth defects, then, are not a significant danger. But all the problems associated with an overly large baby are.

When a patient has high blood sugar levels and is diagnosed as having gestational diabetes, the first step is to lower the amount of carbohydrates in her diet. This may enable the insulin she produces to handle her food without needing to resort to insulin. Since the safety of diabetes pills has not been established for use during pregnancy, her only option, if she can't control her blood sugar with diet and exercise, is to inject insulin. (Some experts believe metformin is okay during pregnancy.)

Her dietitian will advise her to avoid most sugary foods (even fruit is rationed), and increase protein. She will test her blood sugar *after* every meal. That's opposite from when most people test their blood sugar. The reason for this change is that she needs to know if the amount of carbohydrate in the meal made her blood sugar go above 120. She even tests her urine for ketones because if she eats *too little* carbohydrate, her body will start using fats. Ketones are toxic by-products of burning fat. She may need to increase her carbohydrates and use injected insulin to keep her blood sugar under control. Fortunately, about 80% of the time, gestational diabetes can be managed with careful diet alone.

Testing blood sugar, testing urine for ketones, not being able to drink juice or grab a piece of fruit whenever they want, and maybe *still* needing insulin shots, are sacrifices that women with gestational diabetes need to make. Still, a normal pregnancy lasts 37 to 40 weeks and the gestational diet and treatment usually only start at 24 to 28 weeks. Most women will gladly do what's necessary for three months or so. After all, Shauna did it for over a year and felt it was well worth it.

Though only about 3% of the moms with gestational diabetes stay diabetic after the baby is born, about 50 to 60% of the women who get it, develop type 2 diabetes in the next five to ten years, especially if they are obese.

Women who have had gestational diabetes should expect it to recur with every pregnancy. They should also be checked yearly for diabetes, and try to prevent it as much as possible by exercising and maintaining a normal weight.

They should also use reliable contraception and be tested for diabetes *before* they try to get pregnant again. Elevated blood sugar can be devastating to the fetus–no matter what type of diabetes the mom has.

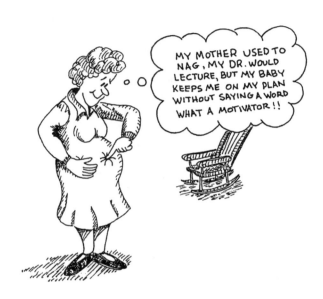

Helping A Pregnant Woman With Diabetes

To The Partner

One of the members of the team that a pregnant woman needs besides the doctors and nurse and dietitian, is her partner. Pregnancy for a type 1 or type 2 woman with diabetes should be a carefully thought out event with weeks of preparation to prevent birth defects. Consistent, responsible use of birth control is essential to be sure conception occurs only when the diabetes is under the best control.

A diabetic pregnancy is an expensive pregnancy. Even if everything goes well, lots of medical tests and doctor visits are required. This is one area where if the mother has insurance, companies are willing to pay to prevent expensive problems. The same woman who couldn't get approved for an insulin pump or continuous glucose monitor earlier, can often get coverage when she plans to get pregnant. Compared to paying for extra hospital days, a caesarian delivery, and birth defects, $5,000 for an insulin pump looks like a bargain to an insurance carrier.

Even with good insurance, a diabetic pregnancy will probably cost significantly more. Couples need to prepare for this so the bills don't spoil what should be a happy event.

To Other People In the Expectant Mom's Life

In the movie *Steel Magnolias* a woman with diabetes has a baby she's advised not to have, and dies of a stroke caused by complications related to kidney failure. If you saw this movie, do not tell the diabetic mom about it or bring up the concerns that were depicted. This case is *not typical* of what happens to most women with diabetes who become pregnant these days.

Another unlikely fear is that a mother with type 1 will pass diabetes to her baby. The chances of the diabetic mother passing type 1 diabetes on to her child are very low, about 4% for those under 25, and only 1% for those over 25–about the same as a woman without diabetes. Interestingly, fathers with type 1 have twice as much chance of passing on diabetes to their children–around 6 to 10%. A genetic counselor can help a family make an informed decision.

If you want to be informed, read anything by Lois Jovanovic, a physician with type 1 diabetes who has had two healthy children, takes care of her family, practices medicine, and writes books. You'll be reassured and you'll be able to pass on the good news that the baby is unlikely to get diabetes and with good diabetes control, frequent monitoring of fetus and mother, and teamwork, the chance of the mother's life being shortened is very slight.

In short, collect *success* stories you can share with your pregnant family member, friend, co-worker. You'll stand out from the crowd.

15

Diabetes Is Tougher When You're A Kid

Preschool Children

Of the 230,000 children and teenagers with diabetes in the U.S., the vast majority are school age or older. Still, a few get it as infants and toddlers.

Remember how overwhelmed John's mother (Chapter 3) felt when he got it when he was nine? Imagine a mother and father of a six month old who will have to do all the diabetes management of their child without the child being able to tell them how he or she is feeling. And worse, not being able to understand that the parents are not trying to cause pain.

Gloria was a year and two months when her mother became alarmed at her totally sopping diaper and bed, lack of energy, and voracious thirst. The pediatrician checked her all over for a virus but found nothing. He sent her home with reassuring words.

The next morning Gloria's mom couldn't wake her. A rush drive to the emergency room and many anxious minutes later, the diagnosis was diabetes.

Gloria got IV fluids and insulin while she was in the hospital and perked up in no time. Meanwhile her mother was given a crash course on what she needed to know about taking care of her daughter–testing her blood for sugar and her urine for ketones, measuring and giving insulin and treating a low blood sugar reaction, and much more.

A Parent's Feelings

Gloria's mom and dad were devastated. Their perfect little girl wasn't perfect. And "everybody knows" diabetes is passed on in families so one of them was to *blame.*

These are the normal feelings of parents of kids with diabetes and these feelings don't go away easily. They pop up at inopportune times, when parents should discipline but don't, when they should say no to an extravagant request but say yes; the temptation to want to compensate for what they believe is their fault is always lurking. It's not a feeling that serves the parents or the child well.

Gloria's mom, especially, felt overwhelmed and terrified. Although Gloria's dad was sometimes there and listened to the nurse's and dietitian's explanations, he was going to be at work most of the day so it was clear who was going to have to do almost all the diabetes chores.

It is still important for a father and other care givers to learn how to give shots and test blood sugar. Not just for the obvious reason that it gives the other parent a chance to be off duty. The more important reason is so a small child doesn't get the idea that there is a "bad" parent who gives shots and a "good" parent who doesn't.

Meanwhile, Gloria was back to her happy self except when she had to have a finger pricked for a blood test, or get a shot of insulin. Her mom and dad *hated* to do these things to her but there just was no alternative. Small kids almost never get type 2 diabetes the kind that can be managed with diet and pills. They get type 1 which requires insulin injections and frequent blood sugar testing.

Managing The Diet

When almost anyone thinks of a diabetic diet especially in relation to children, "no sweets" comes to mind. But their diet is much more complex than just limiting sugary treats. Milk has lactose (milk sugar), juice has fructose (fruit sugar), bread has carbohydrate that turns into sugar.

Gloria's mom will be saying "no" to a lot more than lollipops. She'll sometimes have to refuse Gloria's request for another glass of milk or juice or a second piece of toast. It will be a long time before Gloria will understand why her mother won't let her have another pancake–and her mother will dry a lot of tears of frustration that other moms won't.

Low Blood Sugar

Some children with type 2 diabetes need to test their blood sugar only once or twice a day. But children with type 1 need to test several times a day.

Since Gloria can't recognize her own blood sugar lows, her mom needs to test her blood at least four times a day.

There are some warning signs of low blood sugar that Gloria's mother can look for. They are listed below in the order in which they generally occur:

1. Sweatiness	5. Stomach ache	9. Aggressiveness
2. Clammy skin	6. Irritability	10. Sleepiness
3. Pale skin	7. Crying	11. Seizures
4. Hunger	8. Stubbornness	12. Unconsciousness

As you can see, these warning signs aren't specific only to children with diabetes. Some are normal behavior for babies, toddlers, and even some grownups. Gloria's mom will have to be a good observer and learn what behaviors *most often* are associated with a low blood sugar test result in her daughter.

Low blood sugar is a real worry for a child as young as Gloria or any child under seven. A child's brain is still developing, so a shortage of glucose for brain cells can cause lasting damage. The goal, then, for preschool children under six is to let their blood sugars stay higher than normal (this higher range is 100 to 180 before meals and 110 to 200 at bedtime) so there will be fewer lows.

Eating And Low Blood Sugar

Do moms have trouble with finicky eaters? Does the sun rise in the east?

Imagine the mom of a baby like Gloria who gave her an insulin shot an hour ago, but has yet to get Gloria to eat the second bite of breakfast She knows she has to get food into Gloria to balance the insulin but Gloria is not cooperating. Getting tough is not a strategy she can use very often, if ever. Eating can't become a battleground for two strong-willed people. Gloria's mom has to use all her parenting skills to not make eating an issue.

New insulins (Humalog, NovoLog, and Apidra) have made eating a prescribed amount of food optional. They act so quickly, that they can be given *after* the meal in a dosage that matches the amount and type of food already eaten.

Juice (or glucose gel or tablets) instead of candy is usually recommended for kids with low blood sugar. Moms, dads, and doctors don't want kids to learn that bringing on or pretending to have a low blood sugar is a way to get candy. Juice and glucose tabs are less wonderful. Gloria's mom keeps little cans and those single-serving boxes of it everywhere–in her purse, in the glove compartment of the car, and in the stroller pocket.

Preventing a low blood sugar is better than fixing it once it happens. Having snacks between meals is one way. Especially important is the larger than usual bedtime snack. It can go a long way to preventing those middle-of-the-night sweaty lows.

Babysitters

Another hurdle to get over is babysitters. Gloria's mom and dad can't just call up any teenager to sit and then go off to a movie. They have to find someone very responsible and *train* that person to recognize and treat low blood sugar. Training means not just a 5-minute explanation and a pamphlet. It's best done in a couple of sessions along with plenty of, "what would you do if" questions.

When I baby-sat healthy kids as a teen, if they were sleeping, I did homework or watched TV. It didn't occur to me or their mothers to ask me to feel their skin to see if they were sweaty. With kids with diabetes this is frequently done. At camps for kids with diabetes, counselors make bed check rounds which include putting their hands down the back of kids' pajama tops to feel if they are sweaty. Sweating can be a symptom of low blood sugar. If the child can be awakened, the sitter should give juice. If not, giving a glucagon injection (see Chapter 9 on low blood sugar) or calling 911 is next. Paramedics and hospital personnel can give glucose in a vein to raise blood sugar quickly. Diabetes camps have a physician and nurses who can also give glucose by vein.

Brothers And Sisters

Gloria doesn't have any brothers and sisters, but if she did, that would be another source of potential problems.

Siblings see the child with diabetes getting extra attention and they sometimes become afraid that their own needs won't be met.

They feel angry, jealous, and helpless about this situation they can't control. They also tend to feel guilty because kids under seven or so believe they can *cause* things just by thinking about them and, of course, they no doubt wished something bad would happen to their brother or sister at least once before the diabetes was discovered.

Diabetes is a "family disease." It affects every member. Every member can gain by meeting the challenge of diabetes, from learning responsibility to developing deeper feelings of kinship, and thereby helping to lessen or lose the guilt.

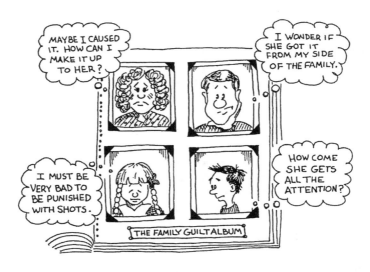

School Age Children

Telling School Personnel What They Need to Know

Half of a school-age child's waking hours is spent in school. Every adult that has contact with the child needs to know what to do if problems like low blood sugar arise.

Nowadays there are printed diabetes information packets for school personnel videos and workbooks (see Resources). Still, nothing beats getting to know the people who make a difference.

School Nurses

It would be nice if every school had a full-time school nurse and parents could turn over their child's diabetes management during school hours. Alas, budget cuts mean three or more schools may share a nurse.

Not only are there days a school is not visited by the school nurse, there are many more children with diabetes now.

Still, you can help the school nurse, and your child, by meeting with him or her before the first day of school. Give her a sheet with emergency information, meal plan, etc.

Ask her to arrange meetings with other school staff so you can explain your child's diabetes plan to them and give them an emergency contact sheet.

Having a good relationship with that school nurse can make life easier for you and your child.

Teachers

When 9 year old John got diabetes, his mother gave written explanations to John's teachers, principal, and school nurse with precise details about John's diet and treatment needs.

Teachers, especially, need to understand the importance of between meal snacks and to prevent misunderstandings, it's not a bad idea for classmates to also know why eating during class is permitted for one kid and not for them all.

In the beginning, John didn't want the other kids to know he had diabetes, so his mother respected that. Eventually, he decided it was too "weird" to have his classmates make up reasons why he had to eat in the middle of the morning and why the teachers sometimes gave him crackers after an energetic P.E. class. So John got permission to speak to his class about his diabetes and he, with his mother's help, repeated his "diabetes education program" every year to his new teacher and new classmates. After his presentation, he not only got resented a lot less for his snacking, but his classmates learned how to recognize his occasional low blood sugar events and to know what to do to help him.

Teachers Are Individuals Too

John never had a problem with a teacher who didn't want to hear about what might need to be done, because every one was willing to learn and help. But some teachers or coaches are afraid of the responsibility or prefer not to know.

Paula had a teacher who didn't want to hear anything that Paula's mother tried to tell her about recognizing a low blood sugar or what to do if it happened. That teacher just kept saying, "I just can't handle this, it's too much."

Somehow Paula got through the rest of the school year after her diagnosis in October and nothing bad happened.

The next year, she got a teacher who listened intently, asked pertinent questions, and made Paula and her parents feel reassured that the teacher would take care of any problems appropriately.

Kira didn't have a problem with a teacher *after* her diagnosis but her teacher could have been helpful while she was getting sick.

Kira says she couldn't go 30 minutes without needing to go to the bathroom. She was so thirsty that after every bathroom break she'd get a cup of water and drink it at her desk. At home, her mother didn't know how often she was going to the bathroom because at home you don't raise your hand and ask for permission. You also can pretty much drink as much water as you want without anyone noticing. Kira was a chubby 13-year old, and no one noticed she'd lost weight. Finally, one night she threw up. Her mom called the pediatrician who lived next door, and who, after a few questions, suspected diabetes. He took a sample of Kira's urine to his office and called back to tell Kira's mom to get her to the hospital immediately. Her blood sugar in the emergency room was 510 and she was so dehydrated from her diabetes that her veins had collapsed. It took 5 hours to get two pumps of IV fluids started and she was in intensive care for two days.

That was 9½ years ago and Kira is fine but she and her family could have been spared some very scary hours if that 6th grade teacher had been aware of and reported to her mother her frequent trips to the bathroom and unceasing drinking. No one expects a teacher to know all the symptoms of diabetes or the scores of other diseases kids could have—just to recognize obvious changes and tell a parent about them.

School Bus Drivers

School bus drivers should be part of the diabetes education process too.

One mom hands the driver a pink sheet with her daughter's picture and how to spot low blood sugar and what to do about it.

The driver is unlikely to face a diabetic emergency during the 30-minute bus ride but she hopes it makes her daughter stand out in the driver's mind and is part of her "safety net."

Physical Education and Field Trips

Special school activities can cause problems at first. John and his mother had to learn how to adjust his insulin and food on the days he had P.E. When John developed diabetes in 1963 there was no way he could test his blood sugar before sports and adjust his food. Today, it's easier to prevent low blood sugar. After the first time that John was excluded from a field trip because a mom didn't want the responsibility for what might happen to him, John's mother would call the parent who would be leading the group, explain the facts, and promise to be available at a phone if help or advice was needed.

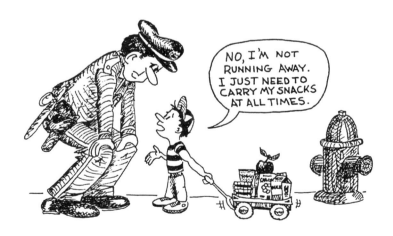

Blood Sugar Goals

Years ago parents of children under 12 were advised to keep their kids' blood sugar higher than normal. It was assumed that complications only develop after puberty and that normal blood sugar would lead to frequent hypoglycemia in children because they're irresponsible and physically active.

Unfortunately, complications *can* start in children. In one 2-year old whose blood sugar (A1c test) was four times normal for months at the time of her diagnosis, her eyes already showed diabetic damage.

It's also clear that kids learn and feel better when their blood sugar is normal. Further, low blood sugar is actually less likely when blood sugar doesn't fluctuate widely. For all these reasons the blood sugar goal for kids age 6 to 12 is 90-180 before meals and 100-180 at bedtime at least 75% of the time.

Type 2 Diabetes

Type 2 diabetes is becoming more common in children especially those over 10. Partly to blame are obesity and the sedentary lifestyle of many of today's children.

If they take insulin or pills that lower blood sugar they are at risk of lows. The lows have to be anticipated so all the cautions, snack issues, and coordination with school personnel are the same as for kids with type 1.

Feelings

School kids need people to listen to their feelings, not so much to get advice, but to really be heard about what's bothering them. And kids are not always consistent. Sometimes they like the extra attention diabetes brings, but usually they hate being different.

Remember when John's mother asked if he wanted his classmates to know he had diabetes? At first he said no.

Most kids complain that when they were diagnosed their parents told *everyone*. And they hated that. Some people, such as teachers, have to know but not every mother of every playmate does, unless she will be taking care of the child with diabetes.

On the other hand, hiding the diabetes, in the fear that other parents won't let the child with diabetes play with their kids, may send the message that diabetes is "dirty" or not nice.

Asking the child who he wants told, in addition to those who *must* be advised, is the considerate route. Don't forget to explain who must be told and why. And, if appropriate, ask that the information be kept confidential.

Help With Handling Feelings

Children with diabetes know they are different but they shouldn't be made to feel that they are alone. That's why diabetes camps are so valuable.

Support groups are another way to give children with diabetes a chance to exchange frustrations and experiences.

Therapists can help both children and parents accept and cope with diabetes. When I asked over 100 people who have had diabetes since they were children or teenagers if they wish they had had a counselor to help them with their feelings, three out of four who had not had a counselor said they wished they had. The reasons most frequently given for why they or their parents didn't or still don't get this valuable help is: (1) lack of money or insurance coverage for counseling, and (2) not knowing where to find a good counselor.

Teenagers

Hormones do not make diabetes easier. The surge of sex hormones that arrives with puberty usually makes it harder to control blood sugar.

Young women especially, notice that their menstrual cycles change their insulin needs. The increase in hormones two to five days before a period usually requires more insulin to keep blood sugar normal. When the hormone level drops and the menstrual period arrives, insulin has to be reduced to usual or below usual levels.

Teenagers need to be in good diabetes control to concentrate in school and participate in sports. Low blood sugars muddle thinking, while highs cause fatigue. Up until puberty, complications are relatively rare. At puberty, whatever protection childhood (before raging hormones) provides disappears. Tight control of blood sugar is not only doable, but advisable. The blood sugar range to shoot for after 12 years of age is 90-130 before meals and 90-150 at bedtime.

Unfortunately, many pressures of the teen years work against good control.

Furthering many of those pressures is the feeling teens have that nothing serious can happen to them. Feeling invulnerable is a heck of a feeling for someone with diabetes who *is* vulnerable to short-term problems like high and low blood sugars and long-term complications like kidney disease and blindness. Many teens experiment with drugs, cigarettes, and alcohol. Teens with diabetes have all those temptations plus their insulin to "play" with. It's not unusual for some teens to be hospitalized for high blood sugars because they didn't take their insulin. Their answer? "I wanted to see what would happen if I didn't take it" or "I forgot it at home."

One 17 year old admitted to our hospital for the sixth time in two years for ketoacidosis from not taking his insulin, couldn't understand why the nurses and doctors were so concerned. His comment was, "So what if I'm in the hospital a lot? My dad has good insurance."

Feeling different is another problem for teenagers. If you've ever been 15, you know what a big deal a pimple was! It loomed and you "knew" that was all anyone was going to see when they looked at you. Imagine being a teen with diabetes and having to wear a medical ID bracelet, and test your blood sugar at the pizza parlor, and maybe give yourself a shot, and risk passing out from a low blood sugar if you overdo it at tennis or track?

There are lots of reasons why not wearing the bracelet, not testing, skipping or delaying the insulin and on and on, looks like a good idea at the time.

Dieting

Teenage girls frequently don't like their bodies at this age so they try dieting. They can get low blood sugar as Kira did from skipping a meal. For Kira who was driving, that missed dinner could have had tragic consequences.

People who have diabetes have a way to lose weight that some take advantage of, to their detriment. If they skimp on insulin and let their blood sugar get in the 200's or even higher, their kidneys try to normalize their blood sugar by "spilling" sugar. The sugar they lose in their urine is full of calories that won't be used as food or stored as fat. They'll also lose fluid in all that urine. Their bodies will also burn stored fat in an attempt to provide desperately needed fuel. They can lose 5 pounds in a couple of days without missing a meal. But the high blood sugars make them tired, a little nauseated, and add to their risk for long-term complications later in their lives. It's a bad idea, but too frequently the short term "sure thing" of being a little slimmer, seems more desirable then preventing possible complications down the road.

Young men don't usually want to lose weight, they want to build muscle. They hear claims of protein supplements that will "bulk them up" so they buy them. Extra protein isn't necessary to build muscle; exercise and weight-training are. Protein drinks and too much meat and dairy products are a strain on kidneys and add saturated fats that can increase circulatory problems later on.

A healthy amount of meat for a young adult is 5 ounces a day. That's about 2 servings, each the size of a deck of cards. Most young men in this country eat 3 to 6 times the amount they need. Teenage girls eat, on average, twice the daily protein recommended.

Life Goals

Diabetes can interfere with teens' dreams and independence while growing up, and eventually as adults as well. They may be discriminated against by prospective employers. Some jobs will be out of reach, such as being in the armed forces. Airline pilots cannot use insulin. Being an interstate truck driver was also out for insulin users (though this prohibition is being reviewed and is currently relaxed for insulin-dependent diabetics who can prove they are in good control).

Some of these hurdles (like not being able to be a pilot) family, teachers, and friends can do little about. But others, such as helping the teenager like himself or herself more, and make safe decisions are very much our business.

Feelings

Parents need to stay involved with their teen's diabetes care and not turn over control too soon. It is hard to know when is too soon, what will be seen as support, and what will be deemed nagging. This is important because nagging will lead to anger and resentment.

The best way to show support is to ask how you can help. If you've noticed signs of poor control (more low blood sugar, more crankiness, weight loss, a doctor's report of a high A1c, and so forth) don't lecture. Instead, try saying, "I'm worried about you. How can I help you manage your diabetes?"

Praise healthy behaviors like testing 3 or 4 times a day. Don't harp on the results, which may be high or low. Remember, it is very difficult to manage blood sugar with hormones surging. Every high is not the diabetic's fault. As long as the person is testing, he or she is demonstrating the determination to do a good job—by getting the information that will make it possible to adjust food, exercise, and insulin and stay on track as much as possible.

Unless they tell you, you would only know what their blood sugar was if you looked in their logbook or the memory read-out in their meter. Don't do it. Their logbook and meter are as private as a personal diary in which they write about their feelings. If you have a good relationship and are invited to help manage the diabetes, you will know what the problem areas are. If not, finding out behind someone's back will not open up better communication. It might make your son or daughter or friend write down made-up numbers. Even a meter can be fiddled so that what's in the memory is not the real blood sugar result. It could be a test made with control solution. (Control solution is a liquid made by the meter manufacturer with a predetermined range. It's essential for testing to see if the meter is accurate. Some meters know the difference between blood and control solution but don't count on there not being yet other ways to "fudge" the numbers). There are dozens of tricks kids use to fool adults. Every year counselors from diabetes camps come back amazed at the ingenious scams they hear about from campers.

Camp, incidentally, is not just for preteens. Teenagers with diabetes can find it enormously helpful in making them feel less alone. Not every community has enough teenagers with diabetes to have a support group meet once a month. Sometimes, diabetes camp is the *only* place teens with diabetes find peers who understand what they're dealing with. After all, only one person in every 600 under 20 years old has type 1 diabetes. Sometimes a teen never has a classmate with diabetes to share feelings with. P.S. Being a junior counselor at a diabetes camp may be a summer job "with satisfaction benefits:" a great opportunity to pass on some of what they learned the hard way.

Parents can show support by watching blood sugar testing, writing down results, and being willing to talk about diabetes. What teens view as nagging are things like being *reminded* to test. So nagging is out, but being willing to take time to be *with* the teen while he or she tests, is supportive.

What one person thinks is nagging, the other thinks of as constructive reminding. Maybe you can make a deal incorporating this guideline: consider the first bit of advice a "mention," the second is a reminder, and anything after that is nagging.

In general, parents tend to turn over total responsibility too soon. Some structure and continued involvement is important even though the young adult *may be intellectually capable* of performing the task.

Also, the kind and level of involvement is different for a 14-year old than it was only a year or two before. Parents sometimes get stuck in a particular developmental stage and try to continue using the same tactics because they worked in the past. Try new ways of interacting with your teen. Just as Gloria's mother had to find ways of interesting Gloria in eating and couldn't take no for an answer, you too, must not throw up your hands when your teen seems to have "majored in stubborn." Try reverse psychology, try counseling, try writing a contract, try listening–again. Don't give up; his or her eyes, kidneys, feet, in fact, very life, depend on you finding keys to motivation.

Peer Pressure vs. Parental Influence

Parents almost always have a hard time competing with a teenager's peers. What a kid has to do to gain approval from his friends can be anything from merely silly, to stupid, to plain dangerous.

What is the "vaccine" that inoculates kids against risk taking behavior due to peer pressure? It's self-esteem. Teens need to start hearing when they're children, and keep on hearing as they grow older, that their parents love and value them so they will not have to depend on their *peer group* for feelings of worth.

When they are older and usually responsible, they should be told that you know they will use good judgment because they don't have anything to prove to anyone.

Value teenagers for their individuality. Remember that they do not want to be thought of as "only diabetics." Kids with diabetes are individuals who have special talents and who just happen to have diabetes.

16

Feelings: Everybody Has Them

What It Feels Like to Find Out You Have Diabetes

Being told that your body doesn't work right is like losing something you took for granted.

The first reaction is usually to deny that it's really happening. It's just too frightening to be able to believe.

Celeste, who got type 1 diabetes when she was 14, says she was scared. She didn't want to inject herself, she didn't want any part of diabetes. Her hospital stay helped put diabetes in perspective for her. Here's her story:

"I didn't want shots; I cried and screamed. There was a girl on my floor who I could also hear screaming and calling out for her parents. I only looked in her room twice. Once when she was screaming. There was some kind of tent over her bed. The second time I looked, the bed was empty and the windows were open with a breeze blowing in on a cold January day. She had had a kidney transplant and died.

"My roommate had cystic fibrosis. The doctors and nurses came into our room often to pound on her back. She was released before me. We corresponded a few times. I asked about her at the clinic, and they told me she had died."

"The third girl I remember used to walk up and down the halls in and out of rooms. She was in a nightgown and pulled an I.V. on wheels. She came in while I was choosing my high school classes for the next year. I told her I had diabetes and they wouldn't discharge me because I wouldn't give myself an injection. I still can picture her face. She couldn't believe that all I had to do was give myself a shot to get out of the hospital.

To her it would be like a dream come true. I don't know what ever became of her.

I was finally discharged even though I wouldn't give myself a shot. They told me that there were sick children who needed the bed. By then, no one needed to explain what they meant.

"My dad had to inject me. I almost didn't let him do it. I remember sitting in the bathroom–my dad with a filled syringe squatting on the floor with my mom. They were both crying, trying to make me understand that I would die if I didn't take the shots. After a few weeks, I did it on my own. And I got on with my life."

Amanda found out she had diabetes when she was in the 4th grade. She says,

"I was really mad when they told me I had to grow up quicker than my friends. I was so ticked off at the world that I vowed never to talk to God any more. One day I was a chocolate addict and the next I was told NO MORE CANDY. When a dietitian told me about sugar-free candy, I was so happy. That is an invention I love.

"I'm not going to lie and say that I don't cheat every once in a great while. But I don't do it very often because of my fear of AMPUTATIONS. That is something I don't want to have to deal with. It helps me resist temptation."

It's not just kids and teens with type 1 that are scared. Bea was 58 when she was diagnosed with type 2. Her father had died of diabetes complications 25 years before, but his was not the only bad diabetes experience she remembers. She came from a diabetic family. Her mother, plus several aunts, uncles and cousins also had diabetes. This is how she felt when the doctor said, "You have diabetes, Bea."

"When I was diagnosed three years ago through routine blood work, I went through it all, denial, a *lot* of anger, depression, in fact, I was in therapy for over two years. I could not deal with it, I was so afraid. All I could think about were all the aunts, uncles, cousins, the people I loved sitting in wheel chairs and how active they used to be. Most of them were amputees. And this was going to happen to me? I'm the youngest, 'Why me?'

"After some time went by it came to be 'Why not me?' With the help of my doctor, I set out to learn. I went to diabetes management classes. I learned so much, but it all seemed to be too much, it seemed out of reach. How would I learn all this? Suppose I didn't do it right? So I took the classes again.

"I joined a local chapter of the American Diabetes Association and that is invaluable. Now I'm Program Director and that keeps you thinking."

Feelings of Denial and Loss

Virginia, was 40 when she was diagnosed with type 2 diabetes. It was very hard for her to stop denying that she would have to alter her lifestyle.

"I took oral medication at first and thought that was the miracle 'cure' and I could continue the bad habits that had carried me to the point of finding out that I was diabetic. I went to diabetes education classes–actually, I went to one class and went home. I was determined that diabetes wasn't going to run my life. And that included all the brownies, pie, ice cream, monstrous steaks done to a turn, baked potatoes with 'everything,' and veggie souffles laden with butter and cream, that I could eat. Yum! Such blatant arrogance!!

"The more I ignored my diet, the worse I felt. My legs were numb, my hands tingled, my vision got worse, and my temper flared. My blood sugar rode the proverbial roller coaster. I had yeast infections that wouldn't quit, burning urination, frequent infections (pneumonia, bladder, bronchitis, etc.) and I was always tired. I'd get up at noon, take a diabetes pill, eat, take a nap, get up and eat, and go to bed. What a life!

"One day my doctor wouldn't refill my pills and asked that I come into his office for a blood workup. My sugars had been over 300 for a long time and despite increasing medication to the maximum dose, they wouldn't go down. He broke the news that I would have to go on insulin and I cried all the way home. I was angry. I was angry at the doctor, at my family, at

God–I was angry at everyone but myself. But this time I went to the classes–all the classes.

"I learned a lot in those classes. I learned that being diabetic means I have to take special care of myself. I have to take my insulin or my body won't be able to utilize the energy (food) I give it during the day. I have to eat right, exercise, and take time for myself, something everyone should do regularly.

"I wish I had known years ago what I learned in my classes. My mother didn't take care of her diabetes and she died from complications in 1984 at the age of 62. Had I known more about diabetes at the time, perhaps I could have helped her deal with her own condition."

You can hear a lot of the loss that Celeste, Bea, and Virginia felt. They felt they had lost their health, lost the bodies they thought they could trust. They lost their uncomplicated lives that allowed them to eat whatever and whenever they wanted and not worry about high and low blood sugars. Bea, especially, lost peace of mind because she knew what diabetes could do to her–she had seen it ravage her own family. Celeste, Amanda, Bea, and Virginia take very good care of themselves but, still, a little part of them always knows that they are at risk.

Feelings about Food

What would Christmas be without cookies, Easter without chocolate eggs, the Fourth of July without ice cream, Halloween without candy, Thanksgiving without stuffing and pie, and birthdays without cake? Celebrations go together with food. In every society food is part of being with people on special occasions. Having to refuse or ration these foods interferes with the sharing of feelings of camaraderie that have traditionally been an important part of these celebrations.

Staying on a diabetic diet means not only rationing the traditional foods that others eat at will, but also dealing with other people's expectations of one's eating. If the diabetic eats the treats, he risks criticism for going off the diet, if he refuses, he may be seen as unfriendly and rigid. A person with diabetes gets to worry both ways.

It's also easy to break the rules of good manners in social eating situations. Some take it as an insult to refuse food, but refuse is what people with diabetes must do. Yet they wind up with "pushers" who insist that, "Just this once won't hurt," or "You have your pills."

It might be considered rude to ask what the ingredients are before you taste something, but people with diabetes must be wary of hidden sugar so they have to ask and risk incurring the hosts' disapproval. Or worse, perhaps hurting the host's feelings by unintentionally implying that the food may be inappropriate or harmful.

They "budget" for treats by foregoing some food e.g. potatoes and bread so they can have a brownie, but have to be prepared for the "policeman" who might say, "You shouldn't be eating that." Usually, people with diabetes say this interference, however well-meant, makes them feel angry, resentful and defiant.

Feelings About Blood Sugar Testing

Testing their blood sugar is rated as the most dreaded chore people with diabetes mention when they name things they don't like. They dislike pricking their fingers and testing their blood sugar even more than taking shots. That's not so hard to understand if you've ever done both. First, it hurts more than an insulin shot. Insulin needles are very thin and short (at most, only ½ inch long) and injections are given in places (abdomen, thigh, or arm) that have few nerves, so they frequently are painless. Pricking a finger with a lancet is a different thing entirely. To get an adequate drop of blood, the point of the lancet has to be thicker than an insulin needle; it's also usually stuck in a place that has lots of nerve endings–the fingers. Ouch!

The good news is that newer meters need less blood so the lancet doesn't have to go as deep. Those meters also make it possible to use places (such as the lower arm or palm of the hand) that have fewer nerves. So testing hurts less, but it still hurts–at least a bit.

What hasn't changed is the pain of the cost of the strips. The money for a days worth of strips could be spent on a lipstick or sandwich or a day's heat in the winter. Nobody likes to spend money on blood glucose test strips so it's not unusual to resent this strain on the budget that most people don't have to endure.

Other reasons also have large emotional components. Some people feel it is a reminder that they have a disease. No one else tests their blood, so doing it makes them feel different.

The results they get can interfere with their activities. A high reading before dinner may mean taking insulin and then not eating for 45 minutes instead of the usual 20. Or they may have to delay exercising because the blood sugar reading is too low or too high. It boils down to not being in control of your life.

Every high blood sugar can also seem to bring one a step closer to severe complications and raise fears about the future.

Finally, many people with diabetes feel that either a high or a low is a sign that they did something wrong–like being graded in school. If a diabetic looks at the results this way, there will be a lot of feelings of failure like getting D's and F's in his or her life. These feelings come up because even the best adherence to diet, exercise, and medication won't give perfect blood sugars.

If waiting for every result is invested with this much negative emotion, blood sugar testing may be avoided as much as possible.

For others, blood sugar testing is actually liberating. It's the key to avoiding embarrassing and potentially dangerous low blood sugars. By testing frequently, they can make adjustments that prevent confusion, passing out, and mood swings that could cause work and social problems. At the other extreme is high blood sugar, which can bring on a sick, sluggish feeling and potentially ketones and acidosis.

To people who see blood sugar testing as liberating, results are not seen as rewards or punishments but as cues to action that can be taken. If it's low, the person eats, if it's high but not too high, exercise can lower it. A quick look in the log book, can give a clue as to why it went high or low, so whatever it was may be avoided or compensated for next time.

When blood sugar testing is looked at as a useful tool, even the discomfort of sore fingers becomes less important. People who test often say it gets to be like flossing and tooth brushing. You do it because it's good for you and it's just another healthy habit.

Feelings About Injecting Insulin

Injecting insulin is a close second in dreaded chores. It's not so much the injection as what it symbolizes.

When the doctor first tells someone they'll need to inject insulin, it brings back all the horrible feelings of getting shots as a child. Memories of standing in line and hearing other kids cry, feeling doom descend, having someone grip your arm and then hurt you. And those injections did hurt. Long, relatively thick needles were used and a lot of vaccine was pushed into a tiny space (about five to ten times the amount of insulin that is usually injected).

Even when the new insulin user discovers that insulin shots are not nearly as painful as other shots, they still are not pleasant. Learning to stick a needle in one's own body is very anxiety-producing. For the person with a phobia of needles, it is terrifying. I have watched adults cry and cower at the sight of a needle I wanted them to use on themselves.

For Virginia, learning to give herself a shot was terrifying:

"In my diabetes classes I met a lot of other people who didn't want to give themselves injections and neither did I. I thought I would rather die first than become a 'human pin cushion.' It took me 20 minutes to muster up enough courage to give myself that first shot. The nurse I was assigned to, showed me the proper procedure but my mind (and hand) just didn't want to cooperate. I cried like a little kid; tears of fear and finally, tears of anger towards myself at having let my diabetes go to the point of insulin. Ignorance isn't bliss."

Taking insulin can also close the doors to some types of employment. The armed forces won't take a diabetic, flying for an airline is out for anyone using insulin, and a person who uses insulin can only be granted a license to drive a truck interstate after a demanding series of requirements. The insulin user must be evaluated by a diabetes specialist and an eye doctor that he is in excellent control. Again, there is a feeling of not being in control of one's destiny.

Feelings About Complications

People with diabetes will not want to hear you tell them about your grandfather who had it and lost a foot, or any other diabetes horror story you know. Remember that the threat of complications is always in the back of their minds. In hundreds of questionnaires and conversations, that threat of complications was cited again and again as the hardest to deal with. *Not one person said he or she ever needed reminding.*

People deal with the threat in different ways. Some, like Bea, get on the education band wagon, and learn all they can to prevent them.

Between her excellent control of her weight, blood sugar and blood pressure, and the advances in treatment nowadays, the odds are that Bea at 61, will never suffer a serious diabetic complication. But what if her worst fear comes to pass and she needs a foot amputated? Will she feel guilt because it "must be" her fault? Many do. Everybody goes off their diet once in a while. It may even be a good idea because it makes it easier to stay on it the other 99% of the time. But those "treat times" may come back to haunt even someone conscientious like Bea. She could end up blaming herself and feeling guilty for being human.

Some people believe complications are caused by fate. They think that it's how long you have diabetes that makes the difference not *how high* blood sugar was *for how long* that does it. And until recently, many physicians defended this attitude because there was no solid proof to the contrary. Now the Diabetes Complications and Control Trial (DCCT) discussed in Chapter 4 on treatment, has shown us that it's the high blood sugar that is the culprit.

For the people who think complications just happen like a bolt of lightning, controlling blood sugar and seeing doctors are a waste of time and money. One 18 year old young man was admitted to the hospital extremely ill, in kidney failure. He had not seen a doctor in seven years. He had been feeling progressively sicker for months but he and his parents had done nothing. His insulin had not been adjusted in all that time and, of course, he hadn't had a test of his kidney function. The only happy part of his story is that he had been too sick to leave his parents' home for so long that a kidney dialysis treatment, in a room full of other kidney failure patients, to him was a social occasion–the high point of his day.

But bringing up complications in the belief that they will make someone with diabetes work harder at controlling their blood sugar isn't a good idea. Doctors and diabetes educators have traditionally tried scare tactics to make patients follow orders. It still doesn't work very well. Studies show that people are generally so terrified by the horror stories that their brains turn off the rest of the message. They blot it out with, "That won't happen to me, so I can tune out now."

Interestingly, though professionals told patients and families about complications and how to prevent them, they didn't write about how to deal with them if and when they did happen. Until 1993, when Judy Curtis wrote *Living With Diabetes Complications,* no book was devoted to this subject though thousands of people were and are living and struggling with nerve damage, kidney disease, blindness, impotence, cardiovascular disease, and amputations. The topic was felt to be too depressing.

It is depressing to lose a sense of control of your body, expectations for the future, financial power, energy, and perhaps independence. But it's even more depressing to have your feelings ignored because they're uncomfortable to hear *and* have limited access to the information you need.

Fortunately, there are now several books on diabetic complications to choose from plus the internet allows many more opportunities for sharing information with others with complications.

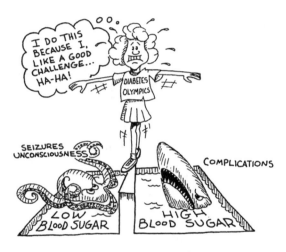

Feelings About Medical Professionals

Nearly every person who has had diabetes for at least five years, has a story to tell about how a doctor or nurse or some other professional has let him or her down. Carrie tells of many times having to educate an "expert" about the disease. One physician said he couldn't understand why her blood sugars wouldn't normalize even though she was doing the right things. Finally, after a year of treating her, he told her he didn't have much experience with type 1 diabetics.

Some doctors (and even a few nurses) don't always listen as closely as they should. It's easier to treat a symptom instead of the cause. This happens when several doctors are consulted but they aren't exchanging information.

Sandie told me she went to a clinic where she was seen by several general practitioners and a foot doctor for her swollen ankles and feet. One told her to walk, another told her to stay off her feet and prop them up, another told her it was heel spurs. Another accused her of not taking her diuretic (water pill) regularly and yet another told her to ignore it, it was just the humidity.

When the swelling traveled up her legs and into her thighs she went to the emergency room. As she tried to climb onto the gurney, she collapsed from congestive heart failure due to fluid in her lungs and heart. The last thing the doctor in the emergency room told her before he had her transferred to intensive care was that she should have seen a doctor sooner and taken better care of herself!

Seeing several physicians is a challenge. Trying always to be clear about aches and pains, trying to understand their doctors' responses, dealing with receptionists, paying the bills, and tracking health insurance payments are endless struggles and very frustrating.

Sandie would approve of Carrie's wish list for what she wants in a physician:

"1. I wish my doctors would consult each other about me, compare notes and make sure treatments and medications don't work against each other."

"2. I wish I could find a diabetes specialist who understood my fears, my desperate need to get my blood sugars under control–and would be willing to work with me to see that that happens."

In a perfect world doctors would send their patients to the most competent professionals possible, including physicians in relevant specialties (such as endocrinologists), dietitians, exercise physiologists, diabetes nurse educators, and therapists, when necessary. Just as important, though, they would also do these two things: (1) praise their patients' efforts and (2) realize how hard perfect control of blood sugar is.

Feelings About Other People's Helping

Fears about what can happen and the everyday frustration of a high or low blood sugar need to be expressed. Unfortunately, many people with diabetes find their family members and friends don't want to hear it. It's more comfortable for us "bystanders" to have the diabetic be a good sport and not complain or burden us with his or her concerns. What happens, though, when your relative or friend says, "I'm going to the doctor this week and I'm afraid of what the tests will show"? Or, "I get so mad that I have to do all this stuff forever and ever." Do you say, "I'm sure everything will be all right." And "Well, you just have to buckle down and do it, it's necessary."?

Chances are, your friend will button up and not say any more. Don't congratulate yourself that his or her silence means you have given comfort. What probably happened was that your friend got the message that the concern he or she had, was not legitimate or that you're not interested. Now your friend or family member feels more alone and believes he or she will just have to handle the feelings without help. That's depressing.

It really is hard for someone without diabetes to appreciate all the problems and concerns that someone with it has. That's why support groups for diabetics can fill a void you may not be able to fill. Still, you can listen, really listen. When your friend or relative expresses worry about the tests at the doctor's office, why not say that you can hear how difficult it must be for him or her to wait for results? Ask what it's like. It's not advice or soothing platitudes that are wanted. It's empathy for and understanding of the concern and fear.

Remarks about the daily drudge of blood testing and shots and diet restrictions are not a signal that you should remind your relative or friend of how necessary they are in preventing complications. Just because he or she gripes about a task doesn't mean that your acknowledgment will be taken as permission to stop doing it. Sometimes, just confirming that the chore really is unpleasant is enough. Consider saying, "You must get very tired of ___. Is there anything I can do to make easier for you to manage all this?"

One of the least helpful remarks people faced with bad news hear a lot is, "It could be worse." To tell your friend Bob who has just been complaining about the frustrations of diabetes, that he could be paralyzed or disfigured or some other terrible thing and that really what he has is not so bad, is a sure way to make him more depressed. Now he has to feel guilty for not being grateful that he "just" has diabetes. Not a day brightener, no matter how kindly or uplifting the comment might have been meant to be.

Coping styles vary. Some people let news sink in and then forget it. Others worry until they have come to some acceptance or decision. Some worry out loud, still others brood. Accepting your friend's or relative's coping method can smooth the way for mutual understanding.

Some men seem to have an especially hard time with a wife's illness or depression. They often feel helpless and inadequate, not feelings many men accept easily. So they'll say, "Don't make such a fuss, you're okay."

If they can't take action and solve a problem they may refuse to accept that there is a problem. A husband might even withdraw and refuse to talk about it. The wife then feels abandoned and angry at him. She may need to stop looking to him for the comfort and understanding she needs, and go to a friend or support group. She will also need to stop blaming him for something he can't handle. Counseling may be beneficial for them both.

Good listening consists of the following:

1. Paying close attention to what is *really* being said.

2. Asking for clarification, sometimes even when you *think* you know what was meant.

3. Reflecting back the other's thoughts with a phrase like, "It must have been..." or "It sounds as if you..." lets them know you've heard and understood and gives them a chance to explain anything you didn't get quite right.

The biggest mistake people make when they are being asked to listen is to think they need to give advice. That's usually not what's being asked for, but there's a lot of it offered. People with diabetes complain that there's a big difference between advice that's offered by someone who knows enough about diabetes to be helpful, and the usual misinformation. They hear a lot of, "Should you be eating that?" when, yes they really should be eating that. But what they shouldn't have to do is defend themselves.

I'm amazed at how many diabetics when "attacked" by someone who doesn't understand, take the time to educate. There are a lot of patient people with diabetes who are willing to explain the basics to anyone who truly wants to learn and not just have his or her beliefs confirmed.

255

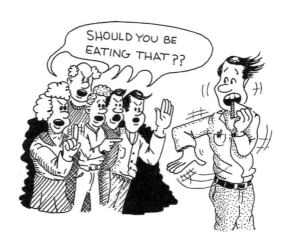

Feelings About Being Made a Fuss Over

People with diabetes are like anyone else, sometimes they are willing to be the center of attention and sometimes they aren't. And being the focus of all eyes when the subject is their disease can be even less welcome.

Sometimes it can open up a discussion about health care policy or a genuine request to learn about diabetes. But there are so many times when the stories are about someone's grandpa losing a foot, that people with diabetes become leery of the subject.

Having diabetes is a bit like being divorced. While divorce does not carry the social stigma it used to, it still is not something you want mentioned everywhere and to everyone. It's not relevant in most situations and neither is having diabetes. The one who should have the say-so as to when diabetes gets brought up is the person with diabetes. Having the right to decide is appreciated and ought to be respected.

Feelings That Family, Friends, and Co-workers Have About Diabetes

Feeling That You're Doing It All

Family members can get educated, supply the right food, sacrifice for the test strips, medication, and physician fees and find that they are the only ones taking the diabetes seriously. The person with diabetes sometimes makes little or no change. The wife may cook the meals the dietitian recommends but the husband eats cookies and donuts between meals. The family can pay for doctor visits and lab fees to the point of hardship and find the diabetic doesn't follow the doctor's advice.

It can be infuriating to do all you can while the person all this sacrifice is for, fails to appreciate it or cooperate. The easy thing is to throw up your hands. The better course is to continue to do your part. It's no different from trying to get a loved one to quit smoking or drinking. It can occasionally be a long process to help someone accept that changed habits will pay off.

This is where support groups, subscribing to diabetes magazines, and counseling can be a help. If the person with diabetes is not following the treatment plan because he doesn't think he can, hearing from other people with diabetes that they once felt this way but no longer do, can be a great eye-opener and source of support. Support groups are where he or she can also hear *how* others met the challenge of doing what needed to be done. And the *how* is very important. Most of us think that a person has to believe in the importance of something and when they do, they'll act on that belief. In practice (and many studies back this up), the more we perform a task, the more comfortable we feel doing it, the more likely we are to continue to do it. The belief in it's "rightness" follows performing the behavior. So doing the task regularly, even if it seems unnatural at first, is the best way to adopt a new habit. You only have to consider exercise to see how this works. Almost everyone agrees that exercise is healthy but only those who have gotten over the initial period of ineptness or being slow have kept exercising.

If the reason your loved one is not following his or her diabetes program is lack of information or skill—books, magazines, and individual and group diabetes classes can provide the necessary know-how. Classes have a powerful effect on changing behavior because participants are encouraged to practice the skills they'll need everyday. Depending on the class, they may write a menu with healthy favorite foods, learn to use a meter, draw up insulin, inject, and so forth. By the end of the class, they can feel comfortable about tasks that seemed impossibly difficult before.

Surprisingly, sometimes hearing someone in the class say something like, "I refuse to give up my regular sodas and desserts" can actually help. *Coming from someone else's lips may be just what is needed to face one's own denial.* Deciding what one is willing to change is an individual choice. But diabetes is serious and requires significant sacrifices to feel well and delay or prevent life altering complications.

If the problem is a more deep-seated phobia or depression, a psychologist or some other counselor should be consulted.

Don't give up until you've tried everything, including sharing your feelings.

When You're Afraid They'll Get Complications

Fear of complications is not felt only by those with diabetes; family members worry about what could happen to their loved one. That's partly what drives them to nag about following the doctor's orders and what makes them believe they have a responsibility to remind and watch and try to control.

Diabetes is more like Hertz commercials than like Greyhound ads. Remember how Greyhound ads said, "Leave the Driving to Us"? Well, Hertz' motto was "Let us put you in the driver's seat." The person with diabetes (after childhood) is in the driver's seat, not Mom or Dad or the doctor; it's just that kind of disease. You can't do it for him or her. If what you're saying isn't working, saying it louder or more often won't work better.

Marjorie was worried about her 19-year old daughter Sandy's over-eating and under-testing. She had tried watching every spoonful that Sandy put on her plate. Sandy retaliated by eating "by the book" when her mother was looking and having candy and anything she felt like when her mother wasn't looking. The blood test numbers in her log book looked great, but the A1c test result from the lab showed she had frequent high blood sugars. Marjorie had tried scare tactics, got the doctor to lecture Sandy, watched and reminded her and got increasingly frustrated.

Finally, she went to a social worker who specialized in family therapy. The social worker told her that she couldn't change Sandy's behavior, she could only change her own.

Marjorie was afraid to stop the nagging and supervising because she thought less control on her part would mean even worse blood sugars for Sandy and sure complications down the road. In her worst dreams she saw Sandy blind and dependent—on her. This made her feel even worse because she wasn't sure if she was afraid of complications because of what they would mean to Sandy or because of what they would mean to her–Marjorie.

The therapist helped her see these fears as normal and not monstrous. When she was a little more comfortable with her fear, Marjorie changed how she behaved around Sandy. She stopped closely scrutinizing Sandy's plate. She stopped making pointed comments about what Sandy should order in restaurants. She offered to sit with Sandy when she tested her blood but she didn't demand to see the results.

Marjorie's loosening up of control was a relief to Sandy. She could stop using so much energy getting back at her mother and invest it in diabetes care. In truth, she didn't feel very well when her blood sugar was high but she didn't want to do what was necessary to bring it down, because to do that would have been to admit that what her mother wanted was best.

When her control got a little better and her next A1c test showed improvement, she was motivated to keep at it.

One day Marjorie told her daughter how frightened she had been and how relieved she was to see her taking better care of herself. Sandy had never really seen her mother's side before. She'd been too busy being angry.

Marjorie did three things right. She stopped being the police but she didn't go to the other extreme and ignore Sandy's diabetes. She still cooked the right food and in a low-key way let Sandy know she wanted to be involved. Lastly, she was honest about her own fear and let Sandy hear, "I feel scared when I see you not taking care of yourself."

Should the Family Change Its Eating Habits?

From the time Sandy was diagnosed with diabetes nine years before, Marjorie had done something else that may have made Sandy's acceptance of her diet more difficult than it needed to be. In their family, nobody else changed the way they ate. Marjorie still bought cookies and sugary cereals and made cakes and pies as usual. For Sandy she bought fruit or products sweetened with saccharine and doled them out in the allotted portions while Sandy's father and brother ate their fill of whatever was the "sweet of the day." It made Sandy alternately sad and mad. It's a common complaint of people with diabetes. They wish they didn't have to watch others eat what they can't.

Sandy's parents reasoned that she would have to see people eating sweets in front of her all her life, so she might as well learn to cope with it at home.

I don't agree. There are lots of things people do to us outside our homes that aren't pleasant. Home should be a better place, a place where people who love you take extra care not to hurt you needlessly. And besides, all that junk wasn't good for Marjorie or her husband and son either, so why not change everybody's eating habits for the better?

On the other hand, some people who have been raised in homes where sugar was banned, say it became such a forbidden fruit that they went crazy when they were teenagers and could eat sweets at will. I suggest a more middle of the road position. Occasional special treats like birthday cakes and chocolate eggs at Easter shouldn't be a no-no to everyone in the family because Sandy can't eat them. Actually, Sandy can and probably should have a small to moderate portion of these things so that she doesn't feel too deprived. Usually, some trading (she can give up the potato, roll, and fruit at dinner for the cake) is possible so her blood sugar doesn't go too high. This moderate policy makes Sandy less of an outsider in the family celebrations and reduces her feeling of resentment. Further, if the everyday cookies and cakes are gradually stopped and fruit is in good supply *to improve the general nutrition of the family, and not because of Sandy,* she won't be the bad guy.

Feelings About Shots and Testing

Friends and family members may find it very hard at first to watch blood testing and insulin injections. Parents may have to do it *to* their child. Not fun.

The really squeamish may wish that these things be done in private. They have the right to speak up. Blood and needles don't have to be out in front of everybody. However, it can be difficult for the person with diabetes in a restaurant, if a dirty sink in a rest room is the only alternative to the table. Consider if it's really something that has to be done away from you or if you can just turn your head away from the testing.

Just the opposite can happen, though. Sometimes a person with diabetes does his own test and several people clamor to have their blood tested too! I've only heard one person complain that testing other people was a problem. I can certainly understand if the expense of the strips is a factor. Once again, the solution is to ask the person with diabetes if he or she minds, and, if you have any reason to think that cost is a problem, find some excuse to compensate by paying for parking or some other diplomatic way of reimbursement.

Feelings About Low Blood Sugar

Taking care of someone who has become irrational because of low blood sugar can be scary. You can see they are getting sweaty and shaky and are confused while they adamantly maintain that they are all right. You know that if the low blood sugar doesn't get corrected, your friend or relative can have a seizure or pass out. At times, help is met with threats or even physical resistance.

One woman told me that she once tried to help get a glass of orange juice into her husband and he threw the juice in her face. That was 13 years ago and she says she'll never forget what that felt like.

It's shocking to have your best efforts rejected, especially when you get a cold dousing. As long as you aren't in any danger, persist, don't take it personally, and don't leave the person alone. He or she cannot take care of themselves, you are *it*. Usually if you say repeatedly in a loud voice, "Jim, eat this candy," or "Mary, drink this orange juice, you'll feel better," you will rouse the person enough so your words and the sugar will be taken in.

When persistence doesn't work, and you don't have glucagon (or even if you do), calling paramedics or promptly getting your relative or friend to an emergency room are your next steps.

Again, when the episode is over, don't take whatever the person said or did personally. It was a sugar-starved brain that fought or insulted you, not the person you know.

Communication Is a Two-Way Street

Just as the person with diabetes has a right to be heard, the friend or family member does too. I recently read an official report that started out, "Diabetes affects approximately 24 million individuals in the United States." Wrong. Twenty four million people may *have* it but many times that number are affected by it.

You have feelings about how your family member, friend, or co-worker's diabetes affects your life and you may need to express those feelings.

Celeste, who has had diabetes for 14 years, just recently learned how much it had affected one of her sisters. Her sister told Celeste that she was planning to revise her will because her three children weren't in it yet. Her sister then told her that when she wrote out her prior will, she had made Celeste her sole beneficiary because if she ever had any complications, she would need the money.

Celeste confesses that she had a good cry after she hung up. She had never realized how her diabetes affected and truly concerned her family.

Be informed, be kind, be patient, keep your sense of humor intact as best you can, and, most importantly, talk about your feelings and concerns. It's one of the keys to making diabetes manageable.

17

Diabetes–A Pain in the Wallet

A short history of medical insurance and Diabetes

Sherill was in a no-win situation. She had a job, health insurance, and diabetes. Her husband didn't have diabetes, but he didn't have a job, either. Four months ago the company he worked for went bankrupt. He applied to dozens of companies in the city where they lived, but nothing materialized. Through contacts he finally got a job offer in another state. The family had to make a hard choice.

Sherill could keep her job with its insurance and they could get further in debt living on her salary while her husband kept looking for work in their area. Or her husband could take the out-of-state job, she could quit hers, and they could sign up for insurance at her husband's new company. *But* that insurance would not cover any diabetes-related problems for a year or two because her diabetes would be a pre-existing condition. During this period, if Sherill had any health problem/condition that could possibly be attributed to diabetes, she and her husband would have to pay for it out of their own pocket. They could lose all their savings, the equity in their house, and even wind up in debt if she required an operation, or a week or two in the hospital.

This is the kind of problem people with diabetes face every day. Switching jobs is a big risk for them if it means changing insurance carriers.

No Job–No Insurance

Switching jobs or getting a pink slip is not the only way to lose insurance. Many companies stop covering dependents when they reach 21. Adult sons and daughters have to find their own insurance or the family has to find a more expensive plan that will accept the "dependent."

A 29-year old woman told me her parents pay hundreds of dollars a month extra for insurance that includes her. She said, "I'm so scared of what will happen when they can't pay it anymore–I sure can't."

Diabetes can have enormous impact on career choice. Many young people with diabetes are counseled to prepare for the day they are no longer on their parents' policy by seeking and keeping a job with the government or some other employer that offers a group policy with comprehensive health benefits. Federal, state, and municipal governments and large corporations have traditionally been havens for people with health conditions or who have family members with chronic problems. Keeping that job can be more important than liking the work. Who could dare leave a job with a company that provided even halfway-generous health coverage and opt for the insecurity of Sherill and her family's situation?

Being self-employed or employed in a small service business is not a luxury most people with diabetes can afford. They've discovered that many small businesses can't afford to keep them when the bill for health insurance comes back doubled or tripled because of one employee with cancer, heart disease, or diabetes.

If the employer can't or won't pay for insurance coverage, that leaves the option of getting an individual policy. If you can find one. Virtually no private insurance companies and only a handful of Blue Cross and Blue Shield plans will sell policies to individuals with diabetes. Getting insurance through a big company may be the only way to get coverage. Twenty-three states have a high-risk insurance pool for people who can't get insurance. It doesn't always come cheap–some premiums are $1,000 a month with a $5,000 deductible. Since there are enrollment maximums, it is not always available.

Getting Hired or Fired

One of the hurdles to getting the insurance is getting the job in the first place. One recent study showed that when job applicants disclosed they had diabetes in a job interview, they were turned down two and a half times more often than their brothers or sisters without diabetes. If they didn't tell the interviewer they had diabetes, they had no more chance of being refused a job than their siblings.

Even if a person with diabetes makes it past the interview, there may still be a company physician with outmoded ideas of what that person can and can't do. In truth, workers with no diabetic complications have no higher absenteeism rates than workers without diabetes.

Generally, one is not required to volunteer information to employers or insurance companies about diabetes or any other medical condition prior to employment. But once the person has "confessed" to one insurance company and is refused, or files a claim for a hospitalization, or after a supervisor is told that the employee must take a break to test his blood sugar, eat a snack, etc., the fact that the employee has diabetes may well be reported to the Medical Information Bureau, an industry clearinghouse. This big computer system will likely be consulted by insurance companies that get that person's application from then on.

If one decides to disclose his/her diabetes early or when it can't be kept "private" any more, it probably would be very helpful to include as many positive aspects as possible, including the considerable loyalty such an employee feels toward an employer, the discipline in life that carries over to one's duties at work, the manageability of the employee's condition, etc.

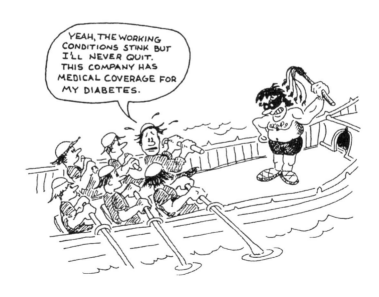

Even If You Have Insurance – Will You Be Covered?

What Medicare covers

Medicare coverage changes over time, for example until recently Medicare only paid for testing supplies if a person used insulin. Now, if your doctor says you need "diabetes self-management training and education," Medicare will cover up to 10 hours of training the first year and two hours a year after. Now an insulin pump may be covered, as durable medical equipment (DME), under Medicare Part B, check with Medicare's main number for your local DME Medicare Administrative contractor (DME MAC). See the section below, Where to Go for Up to Date Information, for website and/or contact details.

Irrespective of your age, what Medicare covers is important to every person with diabetes because Health Maintenance Organizations (HMOs) such as Kaiser Permanente and Cigna, private insurance companies, and self-insured companies frequently adopt Medicare guidelines as their own.[1] What Medicare is willing to pay for often becomes the industry standard; what it refuses to cover is felt to be appropriate for others to refuse too.

Experimental Procedures

Medicare has a policy of not paying for procedures it has labeled "experimental" or "investigational." Thankfully, less is being considered experimental.

Efforts to Reduce the Randomness of Coverage

There have been laws enacted to try and help the situation. Some of the most prominent are:

- The Health Insurance Portability and Accountability Act of 1986 (HIPAA)

---

[1] Self-insured companies establish a fund for employee health expenses instead of paying an insurance company premiums. Frequently they contract with an insurance company to review claims but the decision of what to pay is their own.

- Consolidated Omnibus Budget Reconciliation Act of 1985 (COBRA)
- Americans With Disabilities Act
- The Family and Medical Leave Act

Other efforts to deal with health care expense for specific groups are:

- Medicare for seniors and some others
- State Insurance Pools (only some states have them and they often have limited enrollment)

But these laws have not solved the problem:

In a detailed 2007 study, 62.5% of bankruptcies were medical expense related. Since then, literally millions of Americans have lost their jobs through layoffs and company closings, and so lost their insurance through work or their ability to pay for other insurance. And there's no knowing how many employers stopped providing health insurance but didn't go out of business. Recent news reports suggest that around 80% of bankruptcies are medical expense related.

And in the recent presidential election, the candidate who made solving this problem a principle issue in his campaign won.

There will be new developments about this over the next several years and it would difficult to predict now how things will turn out— and there could be several steps along the way.

Where to Get up to Date Information

Here are some suggestions on some good places to get information on the latest developments:

For national information about new and pending legislation, and about diabetes generally:

- American Diabetes Association (ADA)
  800.DIABETES www.diabetes.org
  primarily for adults and seniors.

- Juvenile Diabetes Research Foundation (JDRF)
  800.533.CURE (2873) www.jdrf.org for Type 1
  and diabetes issues for kids and teens

- The Neuropathy Association: www.neuropathy.org

- Medicare information and issues:
  Medicare adminstration: 800.MEDICARE (800.633.4227)
  Medicare Interactive: www.MedicareInteractive.org
  Medicare Rights Center: www.medicarerights.org

For more detailed info as it might apply to your family member or friend in your state or community:

- Your county or city sponsored diabetes support group
- Your county or city social work department or senior citizen ombudsman
- A hospital sponsored diabetes support group

How You Can Help

Dealing with the health care system may seem pretty intimidating, but there are some very important ways in which you can help:

1. You can telephone insurance companies for a friend, colleague, or relative who is shopping for coverage. Find out premiums, deductibles, and what's covered. This way you will be a buffer and can spare the person with diabetes (if he or she wants to be spared) from hearing bad news. You can pass along only what is useful.
For people who have been refused insurance because of their diabetes, an insurance risk pool may be the answer. For a sometimes modest premium the person receives insurance coverage. The insurance companies operating in the state divide up the difference between the amount collected in premiums and the actual amount spent for health care services to the members in the pool. To find out if your state has such a pool, look in the state government offices section of the white pages of your phone book, perhaps under "Health Division."

2. Giving help in getting insurance reimbursement can be a wonderful gift. It's not only filling out the forms that's a chore, but collecting receipts, talking with physicians and laboratory billing personnel, and defending your relative or friend's need to the

insurance company. Many times a third person can be a better advocate than the insured.

3. If your friend or relative is shopping for a new physician, join the search. Ask any health care workers you know for recommendations of whom they would go to if they had diabetes. Call physicians' offices and find out the cost of a visit and the policy on "accepting assignment" (taking as payment in full whatever the insurance company or Medicare pays). Also ask about spreading out payments for services. These chores can sometimes seem overwhelming. They may make the diabetic postpone getting care rather than have to deal with embarrassing money details.

4. Ask if you can help in other concrete ways. If you suspect a gift of diabetes supplies would be welcome, ask. Perhaps the person living on a fixed income would appreciate a box of strips instead of another slip or bottle of aftershave next Christmas.

5. Last, but certainly not least, write and call your congressmen and congresswomen when legislation affecting diabetes research, treatment, or health care system changes is being considered. And get your whole network of friends and relatives to join you. Some sources say that every letter that is received counts as four hundred who share your view but didn't write.

If you call your local library, and give them your voting address the staff will be happy to tell you name and local contact information for your national congressperson and senators, as well as your state representatives.

US Senate and Congress switchboard number in Washington, DC is 202-225-3121, Mon - Fri 9:00am to 5:00pm, Eastern time or if busy, call your Senator or Representative's local office.

There's a lot you can do directly for your relative, friend, or colleague. And there are opportunities to make things better for people with diabetes in general, too. You can do well by doing good.

18

Do I Have It? Will I Get It?

Do I Have It?

It's estimated that about a fourth (six million) of the people with diabetes don't know they have it. They are, almost exclusively, people with type 2 diabetes, the kind most often found in older adults. If you had type 1 diabetes, you'd probably know it. The symptoms are intrusive, obvious, and, in a matter of days or weeks, cause a person to feel very sick and, without treatment, lapse into a diabetic coma. Here's the list of type 1 diabetes symptoms that was given in Chapter 3.

Increased hunger	Nausea and vomiting
Weight loss	Abdominal pain
Tiredness	Headache
Infections	Leg cramps
Increased Thirst	Irritability
Increased Urination	Blurred vision

The symptoms of type 2 diabetes can be the same as those for type 1 but they are usually less obvious. Sometimes it's diagnosed on the basis of a routine blood test without diabetes even being suspected. All too frequently, however, a complication of diabetes is diagnosed *before* the diabetes itself. This is what happens to some of the six million people with undiscovered diabetes. If there are symptoms of type 2 diabetes present they usually are:

Tingling, numbness, or pain in legs or feet
Slow healing of cuts and sores
Frequent skin infections or itchy skin
Tiredness or drowsiness

These are not the kind of symptoms that send one running to the doctor. Sometimes, you're not sure what's significant and what's not. For example, lots of us have aching feet at the end of the day. When is that pain due to more than just normal wear and tear? Or how do you know when a cut is healing slowly enough to need medical attention? And how often do you have to get a skin infection or itchy skin for it to be considered "frequent?" The answers to these questions are not exact but the rule of thumb is, if it's a new symptom or is more severe than usual, get it checked.

Often, the symptoms of type 1 diabetes are present in type 2. In that case, you'd probably call your doctor or schedule a checkup without delay. It's the cases that don't have these noticeable symptoms that go undiagnosed.

The bottom line is–be alert for these symptoms and have a checkup just to be sure. Tell your doctor your suspicions, and expect to be given a blood test and perhaps follow-up tests if the first suggests that there is a problem.

If the results are negative for high levels of sugar, congratulations. I hope all your future tests have the same good news.

Will I Get It?

You may be worried about your own chances of getting diabetes. Some people are more likely to get it than others. The odds are greater if you have any of these risk factors:

- Are physically inactive
- Have had gestational diabetes or have given birth to a baby that weighed more than 9 pounds
- Have a parent, brother, or sister with diabetes
- Have a family background that is African American, Alaska Native, American Indian, Asian American, Hispanic/Latino, or Pacific Islander
- Have high blood pressure–140/90 mmHg or above–or being treated for high blood pressure
- Have HDL, or "good," cholesterol below 35 mg/dl, or a triglyceride level above 250 mg/dl
- Have polycystic ovary syndrome (PCOS)
- Impaired fasting glucose (IFG) or impaired glucose tolerance (IGT) on a previous blood test

- Have other conditions associated with insulin resistance, such as severe obesity or a condition called acanthosis nigracans, characterized by a dark, velvety rash around the neck or armpits
- Have a history of cardiovascular disease

The American Diabetes Association recommends that testing to detect prediabetes and type 2 diabetes be considered in adults without symptoms who are overweight or obese and have one or more additional risk factors for diabetes. In those without these risk factors, testing should begin at age 45.

Preventing Type 2 Diabetes

There are some things on the list above that you can change. You can do a lot about keeping your weight within normal limits. Moving your body is a great help in making this happen. Exercise does a lot of good things. Exercise burns calories, brightens mood, strengthens the heart, improves insulin use, and increases energy. About the only thing it doesn't do is help you carry a tune!

Muscles that are exercised use insulin better so you're less likely to exhaust your pancreas by needing huge amounts of ineffectively used insulin. Eating smaller meals also reduces demands on the pancreas.

One study of nurses showed that those who exercised vigorously at least once a week reduced their chances of developing type 2 diabetes by 33%.

A recent study (the Diabetes Prevention Program or DPP) showed that participants who received intensive individual counseling and motivational support on effective diet, exercise, and behavior modification—reduced their risk of developing diabetes by 58%. Lifestyle changes worked particularly well for participants aged 60 and older, reducing their risk by 71%.

Another group in the DPP took the diabetes drug metformin, It reduced risk of developing diabetes a more modest 31%. Metformin was effective for both men and women, but it was least effective in preventing diabetes in people aged 45 and older.

Getting a yearly checkup is another way to prevent type 2 diabetes. Yes, I said "prevent." Many people have slightly high blood sugar that rises slowly for years before it technically becomes diabetes. At the first sign of that increase, portion-size monitoring, reduction in fat and sugar, and exercise (that again!) can push that blood sugar right back down into the normal range. Let that slightly elevated blood sugar be your reason to change your ways. It's not a sure thing, but there's an excellent chance (as the DPP study showed) it *will* work, and since exercise and sensible eating are likely to make you feel more energetic and prevent or delay other conditions like heart disease, what have you got to lose?

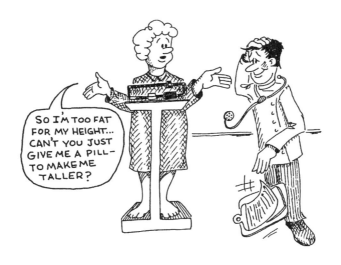

Pick A Doctor That Speaks Your "Language"

To get the most from that checkup, you need a physician who will help you with your preventive maintenance. But not every doctor will say what you need to hear in the way you need to hear it.

There are two general types of doctors. One is the paternal type who gives orders. He or she generally won't explain why it's important—just that you'd better believe it *is* important and you'd better follow instructions.

The second kind of doctor believes in explaining your test results and your options, and then lets you make up your own mind. The theory with this approach is that if you have taken part in making decisions, you will be more motivated to follow through.

Knowing *What* To Do Is Not
Enough—You Have to Know *How*

Whichever type of doctor suits your personality, before you leave his or her office, make sure you get the tools you need to meet your needs. These might include a referral to a dietitian for a personalized diet plan, or a session with an exercise physiologist for a safe, realistic exercise plan. A flippant, "Lose 30 pounds and start working out" is not enough for most of us.

Preventing Type 1 Diabetes: A Research Study

Type 1 diabetes is believed to be caused by something that triggers an attack by the immune system on the body's own pancreas cells. That something could be one or more viruses, cow's milk, or another environmental substance that hasn't yet been suspected.

Several research studies are working on finding type 1 long before there are symptoms by regularly measuring antibodies in those at high risk and protecting the pancreas cells from attack and death. And since type 1 diabetes does have a higher incidence in families with at least one person with type 1, it is those other family members who are being studied to learn more about how the disease occurs.

In another study, participants swallow insulin in a pill form. No, it doesn't lower their blood sugar nor can an insulin pill help control the diabetes of their family member who already has it; oral insulin is too changed by digestive acids to do what injected insulin does. What researchers think it might do though, is be absorbed across the intestinal walls and sensitize protective cells nearby which then look for more insulin, finally settling in the pancreas. There they would secrete a substance that may prevent any inflammation and destruction of insulin-producing cells.

Subjects for this study are family members of a person with type 1 whose blood tests show that the immune system attack upon the pancreas has already begun. These folks have a 25% to 50% chance of developing diabetes in the next five years.

If you have a close relative with type 1 diabetes, look at "diabetes research" on the internet and choose trusted sites. I recommend the Juvenile Diabetes Research Foundation and the American Diabetes Association. Probably, a diabetes specialist will also know of reputable studies. You might prevent your own diabetes.

You Can Help With Fund Raising and Government Funding

Almost all of us can donate some time or money, or both, to increase funding for diabetes research. If you can write a check, that's terrific. If you can't, please donate your time to raise funds or help in some other way such as helping with a fund raising event.

The Juvenile Diabetes Research Foundation (JDRF) and American Diabetes Association (ADA) each have annual walks in most larger communities. Not only can you participate by walking and asking for donations from your social network for each mile you walk, the walks get publicity from newspapers and sometimes even TV coverage. This helps raise awareness of diabetes in a much wider community.

Contact your local chapter of the JDRF or your local ADA affiliate (they're both listed in your phone book). They will be grateful for your help.

Your local diabetes affiliate can also tell you what changes are coming up for votes at the state and local level.

Let your congressmen, and senators know how you feel about diabetes issues. Senators and congressmen notice what their constituents are concerned about. They strongly influence funding for National Institute of Health (NIH), Center for Disease Control (CDC) funding, and other research.

Thank you for your interest in two worthy causes: helping your friend or family member manage their diabetes and helping reduce the burden of diabetes for others.

Recipes and Favorite Foods

Some of my favorite convenience foods:
These foods are usually chosen because they are low in calorie, carbohydrate, fat, or sodium.

When you're looking for products that are supposedly healthier be skeptical when you see claims in big letters on the front of packages. Generally, when manufacturers take out some of the fat, they increase the sugar, and when they lower the sugar, they put in more fat. Look at the Nutrition Facts Label. Compare the regular with the low fat or sugar free version. You could be surprised–pleasantly or unpleasantly.

Morningstar Farms Grillers Original Frozen Veggie Burger (130 cals., 5 g carb., 2 g fiber, 6 g fat, 1 g sat. fat, 15 g pro.)

Morningstar Farms Grillers Recipe Crumbles - I use this in any recipe calling for ground beef. Great for spaghetti sauce and chili–no need to defrost, just add frozen to sauce. For tacos, defrost with taco mix and water in microwave. (80 cal., 4 g carb., 2.5 g fat, 10 g pro.)

Kraft Singles Fat free Swiss cheese (25 cals., 2 g carb., 0 fat, 4 g pro.)

Oroweat Light Whole Wheat Bread - half the carbohydrate of most bread. (2 slices: 80 cals., 18 g carb., 7 g fiber, 0.5 g fat, 4 g pro.)

Dannon Light & Fit Nonfat Yogurt (80 cals., 16 g carb., 0 fat, 5 g pro.)

Yoplait Light Fat Free Yogurt (100 cals., 17 g carb., 0 fat, 5 g pro.)

DelMonte No Sugar Added canned fruit. (Peaches ½ cup: 30 cals., 7 g carb., 0 fat, 1 g pro.)

Herb ox Instant Bouillon - Sodium and gluten free. (10 cals., 2 g carb., 0 fat, 0 sodium, 1 g pro.)

Dreyer's Slow Churned No Sugar Added Ice Cream (1/2 cup: 90 cals, 13 g carb., 3 g. fat, 2 g. sat fat.)

Breyer's Double Churn No Sugar Added Ice Cream (1/2 cup: 80 cals., 14 g carb., 4 g. fat, 2.5 g sat fat.)

Bernsteins Light Fantastic Cheese Fantastico salad dressing (2 Tbsp.: 25 calories, 4 g carb., 1.5 g fat)

Smart Balance Non-Hydrogenated Light Buttery Spread (1 Tbsp.: 50 cals., 0 carb., 5 g fat, 1.5 g sat. fat)

Beverages

Stash Licorice Spice Caffeine Free Herbal Tea - Tastes sweet without added sweetener.

Good Earth Caffeine Free Original Herbal Tea - Tastes sweet and spicy without added sweetener.

Soy Slender Soy Milk - Chocolate, cappuccino, and vanilla flavors. Non-refrigerated. Found with dry and canned milk or health foods. (8 oz.: 70 calories, 5 g carb., 4 g fiber, 3 g fat, 7 g pro.)

Swiss Miss Sensible Sweets Diet Hot Cocoa Mix - (25 cals., 4 g carb., 0 fat, 2 g pro.)

V8 Vegetable Juice - Spicy Hot is our favorite. Caution, sodium is high. (8 oz.: 50 cals., 10 g carb., 0 fat, 2 g pro. 620 mg sod.)

Recipes

These recipes are low in fat and have little or no granulated sugar.

Several call for artificial sweeteners. The advantage of artificial sweeteners like saccharine, Nutrasweet, and Splenda, is that their use allows a person with diabetes to have a larger portion than could be eaten of a sugar sweetened food. Or it means he or she may not have to give up some other carbohydrate food to compensate for the dessert.

I have not included recipes with fructose (except what's naturally found in fruit) because it raises blood sugar and is associated with a rise in triglycerides which is a common risk factor for cardiovascular disease.

Also missing are some of my favorite old dessert recipes that called for frozen whipped topping. All of these contain trans fats (hydrogenated oils). Trans fats raise LDL (bad) cholesterol and lower HDL (good) cholesterol–a double whammy for those at high risk for heart disease. Since there is no safe level of trans fats, it should be avoided whenever possible.

If you're cooking for someone with diabetes and you're not sure what he or she eats, you can never go wrong if you ask.

What kind of diabetes your guest has may make a difference in what is avoided. In general, someone with type 1 is concerned with limiting sugar and consistency in amounts of carbohydrates at meals, while someone with type 2, who is usually overweight is cautioned to limit sugar, fat, and calories.

Diabetes cookbooks can be bought from the American Diabetes Association on-line or in most general bookstores. Your local library may also have a selection of diabetes cookbooks. Choose recently published ones with nutritional breakdowns; they will use new products, and address the concern for lowering fat in addition to sugar.

Bon appetit

Soups

Cabbage and White Bean Soup
10 servings

1 tablespoon chopped garlic
3 cups thinly sliced green cabbage or about 1/3 bag slaw mix
1 large carrot, sliced
1/4 teaspoon ground pepper
4 cubes or envelopes chicken broth (make 1 cup each)
4 cups water
1 can stewed tomatoes, chopped, with juice
3 cans white beans
1 teaspoon dried cilantro (optional)

Spray Dutch oven or soup pot with Pam. Stir in garlic, cabbage, carrot, and pepper; cover and cook 2 minutes, until cabbage starts to wilt. Add water, chicken broth cubes or envelopes, and stewed tomatoes with their juice. Cook on high until vegetables are tender about (7 to 9 minutes).

Meanwhile, puree 1 can of beans with liquid in blender or food processor. Set aside. Drain and rinse the other 2 cans of beans.

Add pureed and whole, drained beans to soup. Stir in cilantro, if desired. Cook 2 minutes, until hot.

Nutritional information per cup:
132 calories   0.6 grams fat
24 g carbohydrate   8 g protein

30-Minute South-of-the-Border Soup
8 cups

cooking spray
2 7-in taco shells, crumbled (optional)
¼ cup chopped onion
1½ tsp minced garlic
1 jalapeno pepper (1½-inch long), seeds removed, minced
15 oz can corn, drained
14 oz can stewed tomatoes with liquid
10 oz can enchilada sauce
2½ tsp ground cumin
1 tsp salt
⅛ tsp ground pepper
½ tsp. chili powder
1½ cup water
1 qt chicken broth or 4 bouillon envelopes and 4 cups water

Optional garnishes:
cilantro, chopped
4 taco shells, crumbled (you may use corn chips but left-over taco
    shells keep better and are less tempting). Use about 1/2 taco shell
    per cup of soup as garnish.
ground fat free Parmesan cheese or grated sharp cheddar cheese

Saute onion, garlic, taco shell pieces, and jalapeno in sprayed Dutch oven or large sauce pan. Cook 1-2 minutes until onion becomes translucent. Add the corn, tomatoes, sauce, spices, water, and broth. Bring to a low boil. Boil 5 minutes.

Serve hot, garnished with cilantro (for a hotter version), crumbled taco shells, and cheese.

Nutritional information (without taco shells or cheese) per cup:
86 calories   1 gram fat
12 grams carbohydrate   3.5 grams protein

Nutritional information per cup of soup
with ½ taco shell (without cheese)
123 calories   2.5 grams fat
17 grams carbohydrate   4 grams protein

Salads

Renee's Two-Bean Salad
16 servings

The most delicious way to get healthy beans into everybody. Better the next day and keeps for days.

2 15-oz cans cut green beans (drained)
2 15-oz cans kidney beans (drained and rinsed)
1 medium to large onion, thinly sliced
1 red or green bell pepper, thinly sliced (optional)
1½ cups vinegar
¼ cup oil
16 envelopes Equal or Splenda
3/4 teaspoon salt (optional)

Mix all ingredients in a large bowl. Refrigerate, stirring occasionally. Better the next day.

Nutritional information per ½ cup serving:
53 calories   0 fat (3 grams if you drink the marinade)
10 grams carbohydrate   3 grams protein

Low Fat Hot German Potato Salad

4 servings

1 pound red potatoes (about 3 medium) boiled and cubed
1 tablespoon Bacon Bits
½ medium onion, diced
1 tablespoon flour
½ cup vinegar
½ cup water
1 teaspoon salt
¼-½ teaspoon pepper
⅓ cup vinegar
Artificial sweetener equal to 2 tsp. sugar (usually 1 envelope)

While potatoes are cooking, saute onion and Bacon Bits in sprayed frying pan. When soft stir in flour. Remove from heat.

Mix together vinegar, water, salt, pepper and sweetener.

Add gradually to onion mixture, stirring constantly over low heat a few minutes until smooth and glossy. Add potatoes and combine. Serve warm.

Nutritional information per serving.
106 calories   less than ½ g. fat
19 g. carbohydrate   3 g. protein

Nearly Fat-Free Mayonnaise Potato Salad

6 servings

2 pounds Russet potatoes (4 large or 6 medium), peeled
1½ cups fat free mayo
1 tablespoon vinegar
1 tablespoon mustard
1 teaspoon salt
1/4 teaspoon pepper
2 medium stalks celery, chopped (about 1 cup)
1 medium onion, chopped (about 3/4 cup)
3 hard-cooked eggs, chopped

½ green pepper, chopped
½ dill pickle, chopped
¼ teaspoon paprika

Cut potatoes in half. Microwave in a little water for 10+ minutes. Test for doneness after 10 min. and every 2 min. Remove pieces that are done. Cool slightly. Cut into cubes or slices (about 6 cups).

Mix remaining ingredients in a large bowl. Stir in potatoes, celery, green pepper, pickle, and onion; toss. Stir in eggs. Sprinkle with paprika. Cover and refrigerate.

Nutritional information per 3/4 cup serving:
177 calories   2.5 grams fat
27 grams carbohydrate   0.8 grams saturated fat
6 grams protein

Sunshine Gelatin Salad
9 servings

This golden salad is a colorful, light addition to dinner. Other fruit can be used, just choose ones that are in juice instead of syrup.

2 packages (4 servings) sugar-free lemon gelatin
2 cups boiling water
1 8 oz. can mandarin orange sections
1 8 oz. can crushed pineapple in juice
1 4 oz. can grapefruit sections

Dissolve gelatin in boiling water. Drain fruit, reserving 2 cups juice. Stir 2 cups juice into gelatin mixture. Chill until of egg white consistency. Fold in well-drained fruit.

Spoon into 8-inch square pan and chill until firm. Cut into squares, serve on lettuce leaf.

Nutrition information per serving:
79 calories   19 grams carbohydrate   0 fat

Side Dishes

Turkey Dinner Fixin's

Thanksgiving and other traditional family get-togethers may be the standard excuse for forgetting healthy eating but they don't have to be. With only a few changes, favorite dishes can be made as usual, supplemented with some tasty, low-fat, low-sugar newcomers.

Here is a suggested menu: *Recipes that are included in this book.

Roast turkey
Dressing (Dressing cooked in a covered casserole outside the turkey
    is much lower in fat–the turkey cooks faster too.)
*Cranberry relish
*Wild rice with mushrooms
*Sweet potatoes
*Sunshine gelatin salad
*Pumpkin pie

Cranberry Relish*
11 servings

An uncooked cranberry relish that is delicious and easy. Make ahead and refrigerate in a covered jar 24 hours to ripen. *P.S. Canned whole berry sauce has 4 times the calories and 3 times the carbohydrate.*

2 large oranges
2 large Granny Smith apples, cored
1 12-oz. bag cranberries
18 packets Splenda

Peel oranges. Place peel from one orange in food processor (discard the other peel) and process until finely chopped. Remove any seeds from oranges. One at a time: process orange, apples and cranberries. Put everything in a bowl, add Splenda and stir until well blended.

Refrigerate.

Nutrition information for 1/2 cup:

49 calories   0 fat

13 g carbohydrate   0 protein *From Diabetes Self Management

Wild Rice with Mushrooms
8 servings

1 tablespoon butter or trans fat free margarine
1 cup uncooked wild rice
4 oz. sliced mushrooms (about 1½ cups)
2 green onions, thinly sliced (white and green parts)
1¼ cups water
1 chicken bouillon cube or envelope
1/4 cup dry white wine
½ teaspoon salt (optional)
¼ teaspoon pepper

Melt butter or margarine in skillet. Add wild rice, mushroom, and onions. Saute over medium heat, stirring frequently, until onions are tender, about 4 minutes.

Stir in water, wine, salt, and pepper. Heat to boiling, stirring occasionally. Reduce heat, cover, and simmer until rice is tender. About 45 minutes.

Nutritional information per serving using margarine:

87 calories   2 g fat

16 g carbohydrate   8 g protein

Sweet Potatoes
6 servings

Sweet potatoes don't raise blood sugar more than other potatoes. This is delicious even without marshmallows.

3 medium sweet potatoes
1 tablespoon butter or trans fat free margarine
1½ teaspoons cornstarch
1 teaspoon sugar

⅛ teaspoon maple extract
½ cup unsweetened apple juice

Cook sweet potatoes in boiling water to cover until almost tender, about 20 minutes. Peel and slice in 1/2-inch slices. Put slices in baking dish.

In a small saucepan dissolve cornstarch, sugar, maple extract, and apple juice in a small saucepan. Cook and stir until smooth and thickened. Spoon glaze over potatoes.

Bake at 375° F. for about 20 minutes.

Nutritional information per serving:
96 calories   2 g fat
18 g carbohydrate   1 g protein

Hungarian Green Beans
8 servings

1 tablespoon vegetable oil
½ cup chopped onion
½ cup chopped celery
1 tablespoon flour
1 cup tomato or V8 juice (spicy V8 adds extra pep)
16 ounces frozen green beans (cooked and drained)
1/4 teaspoon sweet Hungarian paprika
1/8 teaspoon garlic powder

Saute onions and celery in oil until onions are soft. Add flour and stir until flour is absorbed. Add juice and stir until slightly thickened and smooth.

Add green beans, paprika, and garlic powder to hot sauce and simmer 2 minutes over moderate heat.

Nutritional information per ½ cup serving:
43 calories   2 g. fat
6 grams carbohydrate   1 g. protein

Main Dishes

A Burger You Can Eat Every Day
1 burger

This is how you can have burger taste with fewer calories and without the saturated fat, hormones, and antibiotics in beef. Plus, you get fiber from the soy. Morningstar Farms products are found in the frozen foods in supermarkets. Seem too tasty to be healthy.

1 Morningstar Farms Grillers Original Frozen Veggie Burger
2 slices Oroweat Light Whole Wheat Bread, toasted or not
condiments of your choice (tomato, lettuce, pickle, onion, catsup,
    mustard, fat free mayo, fat free cheese, etc.)

Microwave patty for 30 seconds on high. Turn patty over. Nuke another 4 seconds on high.

Grill on Foreman Grill (until light goes out) or in frying pan for about 3 to 4 minutes. Remove and place on bread..

Nutritional Information per burger with bread, without cheese:
210 calories	6.5 g fat
23 g. carbohydrate	1 g saturated fat
9 g fiber	19 g protein

Chili Con Carne (Turkey or Veggie)
8 servings

To be sure that I get the very lowest amount of fat in the turkey, I buy boneless turkey breast, remove the skin, and grind it in my food processor. It takes seconds.

To make the veggie version, get Morningstar Farms Crumbles in the frozen food section at your market. It comes in a bag.

1 lb. ground turkey breast or 12 oz pkg.
    Morningstar Farms Grillers Recipe Crumbles

2 large onions, chopped
1 teaspoon minced garlic
1 medium green pepper, cored, seeded, and chopped
2 15-oz cans stewed tomatoes, cut up, undrained
2 15-oz cans kidney beans, drained and rinsed
1/2 cup water
1 tablespoon vinegar
-seasoning mix- (several packets may be made ahead for future)
4 tablespoons chili powder
1/4 teaspoon ground allspice
1/4 teaspoon ground coriander
1 teaspoon ground cumin
2 cubes or envelopes beef bouillon

Spray large pot with cooking spray. Saute onions, garlic, green pepper, and turkey (if making meat version) until onions are tender. If using Morningstar Crumbles, saute only onions, garlic and green pepper.

Add tomatoes, beans, water, vinegar, spices, and frozen Morningstar Crumbles (if making veggie version).

Bring to a boil. Cover and reduce heat. Simmer on medium low, stirring occasionally, 30-45 minutes.

Nutritional information per serving for turkey version:
230 calories   5 grams fat
26 grams carbohydrate   1.5 grams saturated fat
9 grams fiber   20 grams protein

Nutritional information per serving for veggie version:
195 calories   2 grams fat
26 grams carbohydrate   0 saturated fat
9 grams fiber   16 grams protein

Brazilian Black Beans and Collard Greens
8 servings

This is a healthier version of feijoada, the national dish of Brazil. In Brazil the beans are cooked with pork sausage, tongue, beef jerky, pig's feet and spareribs. It's served with fried mandioc flour (most Americans don't love this side dish), rice, collard greens or kale, and a few orange sections. Good with red tabasco sauce and salsa. If you have it with rice, add 100 calories and 22 grams carbohydrate per 1/2 cup cooked rice.

2 15-oz. cans 50% less salt black beans, drained and rinsed
1/2 tablespoon canola or other vegetable oil
1 medium onion, chopped
3-4 cloves garlic, minced
2 teaspoons ground cumin
1/2 teaspoon salt, optional
3/4 cup water

Saute onions and garlic in oil. Add beans and saute 2 minutes.

Add water, cumin and salt, cover, and cook 30 minutes, stirring occasionally.

Nutritional information per serving:
111 calories   6 grams fiber
19 grams carbohydrate   2 grams fat

Collard greens
8 servings

2 teaspoons oil
2 cloves garlic, minced
1 bunch (about 1 pound) collard greens, washed
3 tablespoons water

Discard thick veins and slice collard greens *very thin*. Cook garlic in oil until toasty. Quickly add greens, stir, add water, cover and cook 1-2 minutes.

Nutritional information per serving:
10 calories   1 gram fat
2 grams carbohydrate

Tom's Kung Pao Chicken
8 servings

This is a delicious spicy Szechwan dish that is adjustable in pepperiness.

Marinate together 3-24 hours:
1 pound skinless, boneless chicken breast, cubed
3 tablespoons white wine
3 tablespoons cornstarch
1/8 teaspoon-1/4 teaspoon ground white or black pepper

Cooking sauce - mix and set aside:
2 cups chicken broth (made with envelopes or cubes)
½ cup water
1 cup soy sauce
½ cup vinegar
½ cup white wine
sweetener equal to 1/3 cup sugar (more if wine is dry)
½ cup corn starch (reserve and stir into sauce just before adding to cooking pot)

Have ready before beginning cooking:
4 teaspoons vegetable oil
10-40 arbol dried chili peppers (Count larger ones as 2. Use only 10 for mild version. You can make dish hotter by cutting or tearing all chilies in half before cooking.)
3/4 cup canned salted cocktail peanuts (NOT dry roasted or Spanish)
1 tablespoon minced ginger root
1 tablespoon minced garlic
16 oz frozen Chinese vegetables
2 8-oz. cans sliced water chestnuts, drained
3-5 green onions in 1/2-inch pieces (white and green parts)
cooked rice

Heat 1 teaspoon oil in a small frying pan. Add chili peppers. Cook stirring constantly for about 30-60 seconds, until first chilis are slightly blackened. Undercooking is better than overcooking. Remove chilis from pan.

Without cleaning pan, heat another teaspoon of oil, add peanuts and cook stirring constantly for about 60 seconds, until first peanuts are slightly blackened. Undercooking is better than over cooking. Set aside.

Heat another 2 teaspoons oil in Dutch oven or large frying pan; quickly stir in ginger and garlic. Add chicken and any marinade not absorbed. Stir occasionally until some chicken is browned (3-5 min.). Overcooking is better than undercooking.

Add green onions, water chestnuts, and Chinese vegetables, stirring between each. Quickly stir corn starch into cooking sauce and add to pot. Stir in peanuts and chili peppers. Stir constantly until thickened (about 5 to 10 minutes). Serve with rice.

Nutritional information per serving:
303 calories   11 grams fat
27 grams carbohydrate   20 grams protein
2 grams fiber

Each 1/2 cup cooked rice has 100 calories, 22 grams carbohydrate, and 2 grams protein.

Poached Salmon with Dill Sauce
8 servings

4 salmon steaks (1-inch thick)
1 cup dry white wine
4 cups water
2 tablespoons lemon juice
1 onion, chopped
1 bay leaf
1/4 cup fresh parsley
1 teaspoon salt (optional)
1 sprig fresh dill
1/2 teaspoon black peppercorns

Mix all ingredients except fish in a saucepan and simmer 10 minutes. Cool to room temperature and strain. (Salmon cooks more evenly if started in cooled broth.) Put broth in frying pan and add salmon.

Simmer salmon over low heat just until opaque. Remove from heat and let salmon steep in broth 5 minutes.

Nutritional information per ½ salmon steak:
153 calories   9 grams fat
0 carbohydrate   17 grams protein

Dill Sauce
8 servings

½ cup hot water
1 cube or envelope chicken bouillon
1½ tablespoons butter or trans fat free margarine
2 tablespoons flour
1 teaspoon salt (optional)
⅛ teaspoon ground white pepper
1 cup plain nonfat yogurt
1 tablespoon minced fresh dill or 1 teaspoon dried dill weed
½ teaspoon white wine
1 teaspoon vinegar
½ teaspoon lemon juice

Dissolve bouillon cube in hot water. Meanwhile, melt butter or margarine in medium saucepan. Stir in flour, salt, and pepper and blend until smooth. Gradually add bouillon and water, stirring to blend. Cook over low heat, stirring constantly until thick and smooth. Remove from heat. Stir in yogurt and dill weed. Stir over low heat but do not allow to boil.

Remove from heat. Stir in wine, vinegar, and lemon juice. Chill.

Nutritional information per 3 tablespoons:
40 calories   0 fat
4 g carbohydrate   2 grams protein

Desserts

Fat Free, Low Sugar Individual Cheesecakes
Serves 12

8 oz fat free cream cheese (brick form, not tub)
8 oz (1 cup) fat free cottage cheese
1/4 cup non-fat sour cream
1/3 cup + 1 teaspoon Splenda Granulated artificial sweetener
2 egg whites
½ tsp vanilla extract

   - Topping -
⅓ cup non-fat sour cream
1½ tsp Splenda granulated
   Cherry Garnish
1 can light cherry pie filling
2 tablespoons Splenda
1/2 tsp almond extract

Blend all but topping ingredients in food processor until smooth. Pour into lined muffin cups (foil cupcake liners with paper inner liners removed are especially pretty).

Set muffin tin in larger pan with ½ to1 inch water. Bake in 350°F. oven about 20 minutes or until tops begin to crack. Chill.
- Topping -
Mix sour cream and Splenda. Spread on cool cheesecakes.

Combine pie filling, extract and 2 tablespoons Splenda Granulated. Place cherry and a little sauce on each cheesecake. You will have left-over cherry filling to use for something else.

Each serving (based on 12 servings) without cherry* has:
43 calories	0 fat
3.5 grams carbohydrate	8 grams protein

*Each cherry has about 4 calories and 1 gram carbohydrate

I usually make a double batch (24) of cheesecakes because cottage cheese comes in 16 oz. tubs. That also allows you to use up more of the can of cherry pie filling used in the optional addition. You'll still have leftover cherry filling. You could offer it in a separate dish for guests who aren't watching their sugar intake.

Apple Coffee Cake
16 servings

1 pkg (8 oz) reduced fat refrigerated crescent dinner rolls
3 delicious apples, cubed (3 cups)
1 box sugar free vanilla Cook and Serve (not instant) pudding mix
1 4-serving box sugar free lemon gelatin
1 teaspoon cinnamon
1⅓ cup water
1 8 oz pkg. fat-free cream cheese (brick form)
½ teaspoon cinnamon
3 envelopes Splenda (or other sweetener equal to 2 Tbls. sugar)

Spray 9 x 13 cookie sheet, Preheat oven to 425°F. Press rolls in sprayed cookie sheet and seal perforations. Bake 6-8 minutes or until golden brown. Cool on wire rack.

In medium pot combine pudding mix, dry gelatin and water. Add diced apples and 1 teaspoon cinnamon. Cook over medium heat, stirring constantly, until mixture comes to a boil. Remove from heat. Cool 15 min.

While apple mixture cools, combine cream cheese, sweetener, and 1/2 tsp. cinnamon. Spread on cooled crust. Top with apple mixture. Chill.

Nutritional information per slice for 16 servings:
80 calories   3 g fat
12 g carbohydrate   3 g protein

Cheese Crepes with Strawberry Sauce
8 crepes

This delicious treat is low in carbohydrate because crepes have very little flour. Making crepes from scratch takes a bit of practice but if you don't want to bother, packaged crepes are almost as good. The ones I used had a mere 37 calories each.

8 9-inch crepes
1 cup low fat cottage cheese
½ cup fat free sour cream
1 tsp vanilla extract
¼ tsp grated lemon rind
4 packets Equal or other artificial sweetener equal to 2 Tbsp. sugar

Combine all but crepes in a bowl and stir.

Nutritional information per serving of cheese filling + 1 crepe::
71 calories   1 g fat
9 g carbohydrate   5 g protein

Sauce:
1 lb trimmed strawberries (if you use frozen, defrost)
4-8 envelopes Equal or other artificial sweetener equal to 2-4
    tablespoons sugar*

Mash berries with back of a large spoon. Add sweetener and stir.
    * *8 envelopes makes a very sweet mixture similar to the 10 oz
    sweetened strawberry "bricks" in the freezer section.*

Lay crepe on plate and microwave 10 seconds to soften. Spoon on 2 tablespoons cottage cheese mixture. Roll up crepe. Top with sauce.

Nutritional Information per ¼ cup sauce:
19 calories   0 fat
5 g carbohydrate   0 protein

Pumpkin Pie
serves 8

Nonfat evaporated milk makes a slightly watery pie. Be warned that no pie made with evaporated milk will be as creamy as what you get from a commercial bakery– they use heavy cream.

1 deep dish unbaked pie shell (recipe follows)
3 large eggs, beaten
1 15-oz can solid pack pumpkin (not pumpkin pie filling)
1 12-oz can evaporated milk
1 cup Splenda Granulated
2 teaspoons pumpkin pie spice

Preheat oven to 375°F.

Combine beaten eggs, pumpkin, milk, Splenda, and spices in a large mixing bowl using an electric mixer on medium speed for about 1 minute.

Pour mixture into pie shell. Bake on center oven rack for 35-40 minutes or until a knife inserted in center comes out clean.

Cool before cutting.

Nutritional information for 1/8 pie (filling and deep dish crust):
283 calories   16 g fat   11 g protein
27 g carbohydrate   3 g sat fat

Vanilla Cream Strawberry Pie
8 servings

1 baked pie shell (recipe follows)
1 6-serving sugar-free vanilla Cook and Serve (NOT instant)
    pudding mix
3 cups fat free milk
1 pound whole* strawberries, trimmed

Cook pudding per instructions on box. Cool 5 minutes in pan, then pour into pie shell. When cool, set strawberries standing up, biggest in center, getting small towards edge. (*If strawberries are not sweet, slice and mix with artificial sweetener to taste. Spread slices on top of pie.)

Nutritional information for 1/8 pie filling and single crust:
179 calories   9 g fat   4 g protein
24 g carbohydrate   1 g sat fat

Double Pie Crust

This pie crust is made with oil instead of lard or shortening. That eliminates the saturated fat and saves about 25% of calories. It's eas-ier to get into the pie pan because of the support of the waxed paper.

Recipe enough to make a pie with a top crust or use half for just a bottom shell. For a deep dish pie, use 3/4 of dough.

2 cups flour	*Combine in separate cup or bowl:*
1 teaspoon salt	1/4 cup milk
	1/3 cup plus 1 Tbsp. oil

Stir flour and salt together. Add milk and oil all at once. Form dough into 2 balls. Roll one between 2 sheets waxed paper or plastic wrap.

Peel off top sheet. Slip hand under bottom sheet and turn into pie plate. Pat into plate and peel off top sheet. Add filling. Repeat for top crust.

If baking without filling, prick thoroughly with fork on bottom and sides. Bake at 450°F. For 8-10 minutes.

Nutritional information for 1/8 *double* pie crust:

236 calories	14 g fat
24 g carbohydrate	8 g protein

Nutritional information for 1/8 *single* pie crust:

118 calories	7 g fat
12 g carbohydrate	4 g protein

Strawberry Angel Delight
(8 servings)

6 oz. angel food cake (about ½ loaf or ⅓ round cake)
¾ cup boiling water
1 4-serving box strawberry sugar-free gelatin
8-oz. fat-free artificially sweetened strawberry yogurt
1 8-oz. can crushed pineapple in unsweetened juice, undrained
2 cups sliced strawberries (fresh or unsweetened frozen)

up to 4 packets artificial sweetener (depending on sweetness of
    strawberries), optional
whole trimmed strawberries for garnish

Tear cake into small pieces in a large bowl, add strawberries. Dissolve
gelatin in boiling water. Stir together gelatin liquid, yogurt, undrained
pineapple, and sweetener. Pour over cake pieces and strawberries. Stir
until blended. Pack into a 6-cup mold or pretty glass bowl. Garnish.
Cover with plastic wrap. Refrigerate at least 2 hours.

Nutritional information per serving:
93 calories,   2.5 g protein
19 g carbohydrate   0 g fat

Apricot Vanilla "Eggs"
4 servings

A super-quick kids' favorite.

4-serving box sugar free instant vanilla pudding
2 cups nonfat milk
4 apricot halves, canned in water or light syrup, drained and rinsed

Make pudding according to package. Pour 1/2 cup into a saucer. Place
one apricot half in center of pudding cut side down.

Nutritional information per serving:
79 calories   0 fat
12 g. carbohydrate   4 g protein

Sugar-free Gelatin Squares or Shapes

4 boxes any flavor sugar-free gelatin
2½ cups boiling water

Add boiling water to gelatin and stir. When gelatin is dissolved, pour
into an 8 or 9-inch square pan and refrigerate until firm. Cut into
squares or into shapes with cookie cutters.

This is a fat free food. There's no limit on serving size.

Resources

Juvenile Diabetes Research Foundation (JDRF)

www.jdrf.org; 800-533-CURE

Find a penpal for your child with type 1, learn what fund raising events are taking place in your area, get questions answered, emerging technologies and other diabetes news, etc.

American Diabetes Association Resources

To become a member of the American Diabetes Assn. call 1-800-806-7801 or visit diabetes.org/membership

Call 1-800-DIABETES (1-800-342-2383) or visit diabetes.org
- Got questions about diabetes?
- Standards of Care for People with Diabetes
- Tips and advice for managing diabetes
- Access hundreds of recipes and a guide for eating healthier
- Learn how to get involved with your ADA
- Shop for 100 books, CD-ROMs, and more

Other Resources at ADA's diabetes.org

African American Program: diabetes awareness program for the African American community. Diabetes.org/africanamericans

Por Tu Familia: diabetes awareness program for the Latino community. diabetes.org/espanol

Awakening the Spirit: Pathways to Diabetes Prevention & Control: diabetes awareness program for the Native American community. diabetes.org/nativeamericans

Planet D: resources for children with diabetes and their families. diabetes.org/planetd

To communicate online with people affected by diabetes. diabetes.org/messageboards

Join the fight to increase funding for diabetes research, end discrimination, and improve insurance coverage. advocacy.diabetes.org

Diabetes Educators - To find a Certified Diabetes Educator in your area: www.diabeteseducator.org

Educational Resources Children with Diabetes:

Milner-Fenwick. Produces diabetes videos in partnership with The American Association of Diabetes Educators. Examples are: *Managing Type 2 Diabetes in Young People, Care of Children with Diabetes in Childcare and School Settings. Children with Diabetes: A Guide for School Personnel.* (Local ADA &/or JDRF may know where these can be borrowed.) Videos on adult topics also available.

Classmates with Diabetes. 10 minutes.
http://www.dhss.mo/gov/warehouse/AudioVisualCatalog.htm

KidCare4Diabetes.com www.childrenwithdiabetes.com

Research

Type 1

- TrialNet Study www.DiabetesTrialNet.org
- Abate Study www.abatestudy.org
- Benaroya Research 800-888-4187 or diabetes @ BenaroyaResearch.org
- African Americans or Mexican-Americans with or without (control participants) type 1 diabetes. Participation involves a one time blood sample. www.t1dgc.org.
- TEDDY Study is an international study to discover the causes of type 1 diabetes. Open to newborns and babies up to 4 months of age. (206) 860-6758 or 1-888-324-2140; www.teddystudy.org

Type 2

- Protege - to study effectiveness and safety of a new diabetes medication www.T2Study.com

Suggested Reading - The following books are available at or can be ordered from your local bookstore or from your local library.

Taking Control of Your Diabetes; Education, Motivation, Self-Advocacy, Steven V. Edelman, MD

Stop the Rollercoaster, John Walsh, PA, CDE, Ruth Roberts, and Lois Jovanovic-Peterson, MD - Practical guidelines for intensive insulin therapy.

Pumping Insulin: Everything You Need For Success With An Insulin Pump, Walsh, John and Roberts, Ruth

Caring for the Diabetic Soul: Restoring Emotional Balance for Yourself and Your Family. 25 chapters by different authors on coping with diabetes, starting a support group, etc.. American Diabetes Assn.

Managing Your Gestational Diabetes, Lois Jovanovic-Peterson, MD with Morton B. Stone.

The Healthy Eater's Guide to Family & Chain Resturants: What to Eat in Over 100 Restaurant Chains Across America, Hope S. Warshaw, M.M.Sc., RD

The Diabetes Carbohydrate and Fat Gram Guide, Lea Ann Holzmeister, RD, CDE. Includes calories, saturated fat, fiber, cholesterol, and protein.

Cookbooks

Month of Meals - Amer. Diabetes Association; 1-800-806-7801
   Classic Meals, Meals in Minutes, Old Time Favorites, Vegetarian Pleasures, Soul-Food Selections

Magazines:

Diabetes Forecast (publ. by the American Diabetes Assn., included with membership) 1-800-806-7801
Diabetes Health (800) 488-8468,

Diabetes Self-Management 800-234-0923

Recommended Weight-Loss Web Sites

American Dietetic Association   www.eatright.org
American Obesity Association   www.obesity.org
Weight-control Information Network (WIN)
   www.niddk.nih.gov/health/nutrit/win.htm

Miscellaneous Nutrition and Diet Site

For a report card on what you eat, go the government's **mypyramidtracker.gov.** If you take the time to fill out the food-intake questionnaire (and it *is* time-consuming), you can learn whether you're getting enough of the recommended nutrients. Also has advice on healthy weight loss.

Glossary

A1c test (hemoglobin A1c or glycosylated hemoglobin test) - Blood test that measures average blood sugar levels over last 3 months.

ACE inhibitor - Angiotensin converting enzyme inhibitor is a type of blood pressure medicine that also helps to protect the kidneys.

Acesulfame-K - Artificial, noncaloric sweetener sold as Sweet One and Sunnette.

Acidosis - Harmful build-up of acids in the blood which can be caused by burning of fats when there is insufficient insulin to use sugar needed for energy.

Adrenaline (epinephrine) - Hormone produced by the adrenal glands which signals the liver to release stored glucose.

Aerobic exercise ("cardio") - Exercise that strengthens the heart and improves overall fitness by increasing the body's ability to use oxygen. Includes swimming and brisk walking.

Alpha cells - Cells in the pancreas which produce glucagon, a hormone which acts on the liver to release glucose and raise blood sugar.

Alpha-glucosidase inhibitors - Oral medications that lower blood sugar by slowing digestion of carbohydrates. Sold as acarbose (Precose) and miglitol (Glyset).

Amylin - Hormone that is secreted by beta cells in the pancreas along with insulin. Amylin lowers aftermeal blood sugar by decreasing glucagon secretion, delays stomach emptying, and reduces appetite. Symlin (pramlintide) is a synthetic form.

Anaerobic exercise (resistance training) - Activities that focus on muscle strength and endurance. They require exerting maximum force for a brief time until the muscle becomes fatigued. Example: weight lifting.

Apple-shaped body type - Body type with most excess fat around the middle (belly and chest). People with this upper body fat are at higher risk of heart disease and stroke.

ARBs (Angiotensin-Receptor Blockers) - A type of blood pressure medicine that also helps protect the kidneys.

Arteriosclerosis - Thickening and hardening of artery walls which reduces the arteries' ability to carry sufficient oxygenated blood to cells. See atherosclerosis.

Aspartame - Artificial, noncaloric sweetener sold as Equal or Nutrasweet.

Atherosclerosis - Buildup of plaque in the inner lining of the arteries; especially common in people with high blood levels of cholesterol .

Autoimmune disorder - Malfunction of the body's defense against invading organisms which makes antibodies that harm the body's own cells. Type 1 diabetes is caused by the immune system's destruction of pancreas cells that produce insulin.

Basal rate - Constant, low insulin output from the pancreas or an insulin pump to provide between-meal insulin needs.

Beta cells - Cells in the islets of Langerhans of the pancreas which produce insulin.

Biguanide - Diabetes oral medication that reduces glucose release from the liver, reduces insulin resistance, and improves cholesterol and triglyceride levels. Sold as metformin (Glucophage).

Blood glucose meter or monitor - Electronic device that measures the amount of sugar in a drop of blood placed on a specially-treated strip.

Bolus - Dose of regular or rapid-acting insulin that is injected to cover food.

Byetta (exenatide) - Injected medication that enhances insulin secretion when blood sugar is high, decreases liver's glucose secretion, and may suppress appetite.

Calorie - Unit of measure of energy or heat. Measured in kilocalories (thousands of calories) but is usually shortened to "calories."

Carbohydrate - One of the three main nutrients which includes sugars and starches. In the intestine, carbohydrate is changed into glucose, then absorbed into the bloodstream and is used by cells for immediate energy or stored for future use. Has four calories per gram.

Carbohydrate counting - System of counting carbohydrate grams in foods at meals or snacks.

Cardiovascular conditioning - Progressive strengthening of the heart, lungs, and circulatory system by aerobic exercise.

Cardiovascular disease - Disease of the heart, blood vessels and blood circulation, Includes heart attacks, stroke, high blood pressure, and blockages.

Cataract - Clouding of the lens of the eye.

CDE (Certified Diabetes Educator) - Usually a nurse, dietitian, social worker, physician, pharmacist, or exercise physiologist who has done direct diabetes education for 1000 hours and has passed a national exam in diabetes and teaching. Recertification every 5 years requires taking an exam or earning continuing education credits.

Charcot's joint - Chronic, progressive and degenerative disease usually of a foot joint characterized by swelling, heat, and instability in the joint. May be caused by diabetic neuropathy.

Cholesterol - Blood fat produced by the liver from saturated fats or absorbed from foods like egg yolks and dairy products which are rich in cholesterol. High levels can lead to increased risk of heart disease and stroke.

Continuous glucose monitor (CGM) - A battery-powered beeper-sized device that senses glucose levels from a sensor placed under the skin. Glucose levels can be checked every 5 minutes for the 3-7 days sensor is left in place. Occasional finger-stick checks using a regular meter are needed to calibrate the CGM.

Control solution - Liquid with a predetermined sugar level that is used in place of a drop of blood to test the accuracy of a blood glucose meter.

Cyclamate - Artificial non-caloric sweetener available in most countries. Not approved by FDA for sale in the U.S.

Dehydration - Serious condition in which the body's water concentration falls to a low level. Especially likely to occur during illness when water may be lost through diarrhea, vomiting, or increased urination due to high blood sugar.

Diabetes mellitus - Disorder of metabolism which produces high blood sugar levels. It results from insufficient insulin production or poor utilization of insulin. The common form of diabetes addressed in this book.

Dialysis - Process of filtering

blood to remove toxic materials and maintain fluid and chemical balance as a substitute for failed or partially functioning kidneys.

Diabetic food - Food that is advertised as being low in sugar but may have other carbohydrates and fat. Cannot be eaten in unlimited amounts.

Dietitian - Person trained in nutrition. A registered dietitian (R.D.) Licensed by the state in which he or she practices.

Digestive enzymes - Proteins produced primarily by the pancreas and secreted into the small intestine that break foods down into chemicals that can be absorbed and used.

DPP (Diabetes Prevention Program) - A clinical trial that compared diet and exercise vs an oral diabetes medication to prevent diabetes.

DPP-4 Inhibitors - Oral medication that increases insulin production and decreases liver's production of glucose. Sold as sitagliptin (Januvia) and saxagliptin (Onglyza).

Endocrine gland - Gland which produces hormones that are released into the blood and which have effects on distant parts of the body. The pancreas is an endocrine gland.

Endocrinologist - Physician who specializes in disorders of the endocrine glands. Most endocrinologists treat diabetes more than any other glandular problem.

Enzymes - Specific proteins produced by cells to cause or speed up chemical reactions.

Exercise physiologist - Professional trained in exercise science who is able to design an exercise program. Also evaluates responses of blood sugar to exercise and assists in education of patients. May be a CDE.

Fasting blood sugar - Sugar concentration in the blood when no food has been eaten for 8 hours or more. A normal value is 70-99 mg/dl, pre-diabetes is 100-125, diabetes is 126 or more.

Fat - One of the three classes of energy-producing nutrients including oils, butter, meat, etc. Has nine calories per gram.

Fiber - Largely indigestible parts of plants. May help lower cholesterol and blood sugar and promote better intestinal function. Foods high in fiber include whole grain breads and cereals, whole fruits, and dried beans.

Fructose - A sugar found in fruit that causes less rise in blood sugar when used instead of table sugar to sweeten foods. Has been found along with table sugar to increase levels of triglycerides.

Gangrene - Death of tissue caused by insufficient blood supply. May require amputation of the affected part of the body.

Gestational diabetes - Diabetes that occurs during pregnancy. It is caused by hormonal changes that result in the body requiring more insulin than can be naturally produced. Diet and sometimes insulin, are necessary, to prevent the birth of a dangerously large baby or a premature birth.

Glaucoma - Eye disorder in which increased pressure inside the eye can damage the optic nerve, resulting in blindness. Early diagnosis and treatment are essential.

Glucagon - Hormone produced by the pancreas. When blood sugar levels get low, it is released, stimulating the release of glucose from the liver. An injectable form is available by prescription for correcting low blood sugar of someone who is unconscious or having seizures.

Glucose - Form of sugar most used by cells for energy. Ninety percent of carbohydrates are changed into glucose.

Glucose gel - Glucose preparation in a gel form. Usually sold in tubes that hold 15 grams glucose. The contents are squeezed into the mouth to correct a low blood sugar.

Glucose tablet - Tablet that contains 4 or 5 grams glucose. Three or four are chewed when blood sugar is too low.

Glycemic index - List of different foods' effect on blood sugar compared with glucose or white bread.

Glycogen - Form of carbohydrate stored in the liver and muscles. It can be converted back into glucose when needed.

Glycohemoglobin - Portions of a red blood cell's hemoglobin that collect sugar molecules. Measurement of glycohemoglobin indicates the blood sugar level high over last three months. Also A1c.

Glycosylated hemoglobin test - See glycohemoglobin, hemoglobin A1c.

Gram - Unit of weight in the metric system. A penny weighs 3 grams. Dietary fat, protein, and carbohydrate are measured in grams.

HDL (high density lipoprotein) - "Good" type of cholesterol. A higher proportion of HDL seems to protect against cardiovascular disease.

Heart attack - Blockage of blood supply to the heart that results in damage to the heart muscle.

Hemoglobin A1c - Portion of the hemoglobin of the red blood cell that collects sugar molecules. Same as glycosylated hemoglobin, glycohemoglobin, and A1c.

High blood sugar (hyperglycemia) - Higher than normal amount of sugar in the blood.

Honeymoon phase - Temporary period when a person with newly diagnosed type 1 diabetes may need little or no injected insulin because their own insulin-producing cells have temporarily resumed functioning.

Hormone - Chemical produced by a gland which is released into the blood stream. Insulin is a hormone.

Hydrogenated fat - Oil or fat that has had hydrogen atoms added to it through a chemical process to make it more solid. Hydrogenating a vegetable oil produces harmful trans fatty acids. (See trans fatty acids.)

Hyperbaric chamber - Compartment which contains a higher than normal atmospheric pressure. This allows more oxygen to be carried by the blood and can by useful in the treatment of gangrene. Also used to treat divers for the bends.

Hyperglycemia (High blood sugar) - Higher than normal amount of sugar in the blood.

Hyperosmotic coma - A coma caused by very high blood sugar resulting in serious dehydration. May occur in someone with type 2 diabetes under the same conditions that would cause keto-acidosis in someone with type 1.

Hypertension (high blood pressure) - Higher than normal blood pressure within the arteries. A reading of 120/80 is now considered prehypertension. High blood pressure raises risk of heart attacks, strokes, blindness, and kidney damage.

Hypoglycemia (low blood sugar) - Lower than normal amount of sugar in the blood. Below 60 is usually considered low and *requires* treatment with 15 grams of glucose tablets or gel, or a sugary food or beverage.

Impotence or **Impotency** - Inability to achieve or maintain an erection.

Insoluble fiber - Part of plant (such as wheat bran) that does not dissolve in water and is not digested.

Insulin - Hormone produced by beta cells in the pancreas which allows glucose to enter cells.

Insulin-dependent diabetes - (type 1 or juvenile-onset) Diabetes which usually occurs before 20. Is brought on by the complete destruction of the insulin-producing cells in the pancreas. Treatment requires insulin replacement by injection.

Insulin pen - A device resembling a pen used to hold and inject insulin.

Insulin pump - Beeper-sized battery-powered device which delivers insulin from a cartridge through a tube placed under the skin for 3 days at a time. A computer programmed by the wearer regulates the delivery of small continuous basal amounts between meals and larger bolus amounts at meals and snacks.

Insulin receptor - Chemical "locks" on cells that react to insulin, allowing sugar to enter the cell. Malfunction of receptors results in insulin resistance, a cause of sugar accumulating in the blood in type 2 diabetes.

Insulin resistance - Diminished ability of cells to respond to the action of insulin in promoting the transport of glucose from blood into cells in type 2 diabetes. Often seen in metabolic syndrome, obesity, pregnancy, infection or severe illness, stress, and during steroid use.

Intermediate-acting insulin - Intermediate-acting insulin starts working in 2-4 hours, has a peak of action between 6 and 12 hours, and lasts for about 12 -18 hours. (See NPH.)

Intravenous (IV) fluids - Sterile fluids given through a needle or catheter into a vein.

Islets of Langerhans - Clusters of cells in the pancreas that contain alpha cells (produce glucagon) and beta cells (produce insulin and amylin) that regulate blood sugar.

Ketoacidosis - Abnormal acid condition caused by the accumulation of ketones which are produced when there is insufficient insulin present in the body for glucose to be used for energy. The use of fat as an emergency energy source, produces toxic ketones. This can result in dehydration and chemical and fluid imbalances which can be fatal if not treated.

Ketones - By-products of the use of fat as an energy source when insulin is not available. Test strips are sold over the counter. (See ketoacidosis, above.)

Ketonuria - Presence of ketones in urine. Detected with test strips sold over the counter. Moderate to large amounts may indicate ketoacidosis.

Kidneys - Organs which filter the blood, regulate fluid and salt balance, remove toxins and produce urine.

Lactose - Sugar found naturally in milk.

Laser - Device that produces a concentrated beam of light. It is used in the treatment of diabetic retinopathy to prevent bleeding from weak blood vessels in the interior of the eyes. It is also used to reattach the retina if torn.

Lancets - Small, short "needles" used to puncture skin when doing a blood test.

Liver - Organ which manufactures and regulates level of many of the body's chemicals. One of its functions is the storage of glucose when it is not needed, and its reformation from glycogen and protein. Releases glucose when needed to raise blood sugar.

LDL - Low density lipoprotein, also called "bad" cholesterol. High level of LDL cholesterol in the blood increases risk of heart disease and strokes.

Long-acting insulin - Basal insulin. Glargine (Lantus) and detemir (Levemir) start to work about 2 to 4 hours after injection and may last up to 24 hours. They have little or no peak so lows are less likely unless dose is excessive.

Low blood sugar (hypoglycemia) - Lower than normal glucose in the blood. Below 60 is usually considered low and generally *requires* treatment.

Meal plan - Personalized eating plan which includes quantity, types of foods, and timing. Age, weight, medication, activity, and other factors influence the three components.

Medical identification - Bracelet, anklet, or necklace which identifies the wearer as a diabetic. Some describe treatment or give a toll-free phone number which can be called for user's emergency medical information.

Meglitinides - Oral medications that increase insulin production. Sold as nateglinide (Starlix) and repaglinide (Prandin).

Metabolic syndrome - A clustering of risk factors that include insulin resistance, high blood pressure, cholesterol abnormalities, and an increased risk of clotting. Patients are often overweight or obese.

Metabolism - Sum of all the chemical changes that take place in the body. Metabolism of food refers to how food is broken down into smaller parts as when some of a potato becomes sugar in the blood. It also refers to the opposite process–taking smaller chemical units like sugar and making them into large units such as fat tissue.

Metformin (Glucophage) - Diabetes pill that reduces glucose release from the liver, reduces insulin resistance, and improves cholesterol and triglyceride levels.

Microalbumin - Urine test for tiny amounts of protein. It's presence may signal early kidney disease.

Milligram (mg) - Unit of weight equal to one-thousandth of a gram. Common unit in measuring medications, cholesterol, blood sugar, etc..

Monounsaturated fat - Fats that seem not to raise LDL (bad) cholesterol. Monounsaturated oils include olive oil and canola oil.

Neonatologist - Physician who specializes in the care of newborn babies.

Nephropathy - Kidney disease.

Neuropathy - Damage to the nerves. Almost any part of the body can be affected by this complication of diabetes. Symptoms in arms and legs include numbness, tingling, pain, and coldness.

Normal blood sugar - Measured in milligrams per deciliter (mg/dl). What is considered normal depends on whether person has recently eaten or has fasted. (See fasting blood sugar and postprandial blood sugar.)

NPH insulin - Intermediate-acting insulin which starts working in 2 to 4 hours, has a peak of action between 6 and 12 hours, and lasts for about 12 to 18 hours. The letters NPH stand for neutral protamine Hagedorn. Neutral, because it is neither chemically an acid nor a base, protamine (now isophane), which is added to extend the time it takes to be absorbed, and Hagedorn, the name of the inventor.

Obesity - Condition of having too much body fat. Usually a person must be at least 20% over maximum desirable weight to be considered obese. Obesity is present in about 80% of people who get type 2 diabetes.

Ophthalmologist - Physician (MD) who specializes in treating diseases of the eyes including performing surgery and laser therapy.

Optometrist (doctor of optometry or O.D.) - Health care professional (not an MD) who is trained to examine and diagnose eye diseases such as glaucoma, cataracts and retinal diseases and, in certain states in the U.S., .to treat them; to examine, diagnose, and treat visual conditions such as nearsightedness, and fit eye glasses and contact lenses.

Oral diabetes pills - Medications which may improve blood sugar levels. Not oral insulin.

Pancreas - Abdominal organ which produces three hormones: insulin, glucagon, and amylin. The pancreas also produces digestive enzymes.

Pancreatitis - Inflammation of the pancreas gland which may result in damage. Occasionally, some or all of the gland must be surgically removed resulting in a shortage or complete lack of insulin, glucagon, and pancreatic digestive enzymes.

Pear-shaped body type - Body type with excess fat below the waist resulting in a pear-shape. Fat in the thighs and buttocks is less likely to result in heart disease and strokes than fat around and above the waist.

Pediatrician - Physician that specializes in the physical development and medical care of children.

Plaque - Fatty deposit on the inside of artery walls which results in a narrowing which can lead to an inadequate blood supply in the area the artery supplies. Plaque is formed from LDL cholesterol and other materials. Eventually plaque can thicken until it blocks the vessel or a piece can break off, causing blockage somewhere else.

Podiatrist - A doctor (although not an MD) who specializes in the prevention and treatment of foot disorders including foot ulcers and foot infections. Is qualified to perform surgery for foot conditions.

Polyunsaturated oil - Thought to be less likely to cause clogged arteries than solid (saturated) fats. Polyunsaturated oils include corn, soybean, and safflower oils.

Postprandial - Following a meal. Postprandial blood sugar testing (2 hours after the first bite) is recommended to learn how a particular meal affected blood sugar. Recommended level is 140-180 mg/dl.

Prediabetes (formerly called impaired glucose tolerance and impaired fasting glucose) - Occurs when blood sugar is higher than normal but not yet high enough for a diagnosis of diabetes. (See fasting diabetes.) People with pre-diabetes are at higher risk of cardiovascular disease compared to people with normal blood sugar and are at high risk for type 2 diabetes.

Preeclampsia - Serious condition of pregnancy characterized by increased blood pressure, headaches, fluid retention, nausea and vomiting, abdominal pain, visual disturbances, and protein in the urine.

Preeclampsia is more frequent in women with diabetes. It may lead to the more serious condition, eclampsia which can cause seizures and may require emergency delivery to save the mother and baby.

Proliferative retinopathy - Serious diabetic complication of the retina of the eyes. Laser treatment is frequently successful in preventing progression to blindness.

Protein - One of three main nutrients. Found in dairy foods, meat, fish, and beans. Protein is primarily used to build tissue. Excess protein is turned into fat. Protein has 4 calories per gram.

Rapid-acting insulin - Insulin that starts working in about 15 minutes, peaks in 1 or 2 hours after injection and lasts between 3 and 4 hours. Ideal for before-meal doses. Rapid-acting insulins include: Aspart (Novalog), Glulisine (Apidra), and lispro (Humalog).

Regular insulin - Short-acting as opposed to rapid-acting because it takes a longer time to work than rapid-acting insulin. Begins to act in 30 minutes, peaks 2 to 4 hours later, and lasts up to 8 hours.

Retina - The light-sensitive

tissue lining the interior of the eye. It contains special nerve calls which convert light energy into nerve impulses. (See proliferative retinopathy)

Retinopathy - Any disease of the retina. Background retinopathy does not usually impair vision but shows that diabetic changes are occurring. More serious are preproliferative and proliferative retinopathy.

Saccharin - An artificial sweetener that has no calories. Sold as Sweet'N Low, Sugar Twin, and Necta Sweet.

Saturated fat - Fats which are solid at room temperature. These tend to contribute more to plaque formation in arteries which may lead to cardiovascular disease. Daily limit recommended for diabetics and those with cardiovascular disease risk factors is less than 7% of total calories. Saturated fat is listed on Nutrition Facts labels under Total Fat.

Simple carbohydrate - See sugar.

Soluble fiber - Part of plant foods (beans, oats, apples, etc.) that forms a gel when mixed with a liquid. Improves digestion, blood cholesterol level and slows absorption of sugar from the intestine.

Stevia - Herb that is 30 times sweeter than sugar. Long popular in South America and Japan. Highly processed form (rebaudioside) approved by FDA for use in foods in 2008. Sold as TruVia and PureVia.

Subcutaneous tissue - Fatty layer below the skin into which insulin is injected.

Sucralose - Noncaloric artificial sweetener. Sold as Splenda.

Sucrose - Table sugar, beet sugar, cane sugar. Is used to make granulated, powdered, and brown sugars.

Sugar - Simple form of carbohydrate. Different types of sugar include: fructose, galactose, glucose, lactose, maltose, sucrose, and xylose.

Sugar-free - Term used by food processors which may mean it does not contain sucrose (table sugar) but may contain any of several other forms of sugar. Does *not* mean it is carbohydrate-free or glucose-free.

Sulfonylureas - Diabetes pills which lower blood sugar by stimulating insulin production. They are not an oral form of insulin. May cause low blood sugar and weight gain. Includes glimepiride (Amaryl), glipizide

(Glucotrol), glyburide (Micronase, DiaBeta).

Symlin (pramlintide acetate) - Injected medication that helps suppress appetite and lowers high blood sugar after meals.

Target range - An effective exercise exertion level. Low intensity = less than 50% maximal heart rate; moderate-intensity = 50- 70% of maximal heart rate. Vigorous exercise generally = about 70 to 85% maximum heart rate.

Thiazolidinediones (TZDs or glitazones) - Oral medication that decreases insulin resistance. Sold as pioglitazone (Actos) and rosiglitazone (Avandia).

Trans fat or trans fatty acids - Harmful fat that results when vegetable oils are hydrogenated. Has been shown to raise the risk of heart disease by raising levels of LDL cholesterol and lowering HDL choleserol. No amount is considered safe.

Triglycerides - Lipids (fat-like substances) carried through the bloodstream to the tissues. High levels increase heart disease and stroke risk.

Type 1 diabetes (insulin dependent or juvenile-onset diabetes) - Type of diabetes which usually occurs before the age of 20. Is brought on by the complete destruction of the insulin-producing cells in the pancreas. Treatment requires insulin, diet, and exercise.

Type 1½ diabetes (latent auto-immune diabetes in adults [LADA]) - Has features of type 1 and type 2. Treatment eventually requires insulin, though pills may be possible for a few months or even a year or two. Not a common form of diabetes.

Type 2 diabetes (non-insulin dependent or adult-onset diabetes) - Type of diabetes which usually occurs after age 40. Over 90% of people with diabetes have type 2. Treatment includes diet, exercise, and may require oral medication and/or insulin.

Units - How insulin is prescribed and measured. One cubic centimeter (cc) of insulin usually has 100 units. There is a concentrated form of insulin that has 500 units in one cc.

Unsaturated fat - Oil that is not saturated or solid. Considered to be less harmful than saturated fat. Substituting saturated fats with unsaturated fats helps to lower levels of LDL (bad) cholesterol. Includes monounsaturated and polyunsaturated oils.

Index

acesulfame-K 109
acidosis *see also* ketoacidosis
adrenaline 29, 139
aerobic exercise 192
alcohol 106, 119, 120, 138, 214
alpha cells
Americans With Disabilities Act 267
amputation 162
anaerobic exercise 192
apple-shaped body 79
arteriosclerosis
artificial sweeteners 108-109
aspartame 109
aspirin 67
baby sitters 233
basal rate 61
beta cells
blood glucose testing 42, 59
    advantages 38, 43
    cost 45
    disadvantages 69-72
    frequency 44
    meters 59-60, 65, 248
    recording results 57
    time of test 69
body shape 79
bolus 62
books 318-319
calorie 78
carbohydrate 76, 79-81
cardiovascular conditioning 188
cardiovascular disease 168
cataract 166
certified diabetes educator 55, 82
children
    preschool 230
        baby sitters233
        blood sugar goals 232
        brothers and sisters 233

diet 231
    low blood sugar 232
    parents' feelings 25,231
school age children
    blood sugar goals 238
    feelings 238, 239
    informational kit ordering 318
    PE and field trips 237
    school bus driver 237
    school nurse 235
    school personnel 234
    teachers 235-236
teens *see* teenagers
cholesterol 67
    reducing in diet 85
    restaurant meals 125, 127
cookbooks 108, 117, 319
complications 48
    eye 48, 164, 165
    feet and legs 162
    heart and circulatory system 168
    impotence 172
    kidney disease 48, 166
    nerve damage 48, 162-163
    prevention 67, 169, 174
        how to help 180
        how not to help 179
continuous glucose sensors 60
control solution for meters 242
costs *see* specific item
    how to help 238
cyclamate 109
dentist 54
dehydration 154-161
diabetes
    causes 28
    classes 16, 257
    cure 31
    explained 16, 25

gestational *see* pregnancy
mellitus 16
types 11, 28
prevention 272
Diabetes Control and Complications
Trial 47
diabetic vs person with   diabetes 13
dialysis *see also* kidney disease 167
dietetic food 93
dietitian 82
digestive enzymes 17
dining out 119
alcohol 120
breakfast 123
Chinese 122
coffee shop breakfast 123
fast food 123
foods to choose 130
foods to limit 130
French 127
fried chicken 125
Indian 122
Italian 127
Japanese 122
menus 129
ask questions 128
substitutions 128
Mexican 122
salad bars 124, 125
sandwiches 124
scheduling a time 119, 121
seafood 126
soup 131
steak 125
Thai 122
vegetarian 126
Vietnamese 122
education
classes 16, 257
support groups 254-255
employment 263

endocrinologist 40
enzymes 17
exercise
aerobic vs anaerobic 192
aerobic target range 195-197
benefits 187
exercise machines 200
fluid replacement 205
goals 206
intensity 194
mall walking 208
medical identification 152
myths 201
pedometer 204
personal trainer   199
physical education in school 237
physiologist 55
pulse 195
rewards 206
risks 184
general 194
with type 1   186
tapes 207
time 193
trainer, personal 199
tips 203
weight loss 197
weight-training 198
Wii   207
Fam. & Med'l Leave Act   267
fat   *see* food
feelings
blood sugar testing 248
complications   250
denial and loss 246
diagnosis 244
family fears 25, 258
family doing it all 256
food, about 247
insulin injections 249
listening 255

315

low blood sugar 261
medical professionals 252
fiber   98
food
   beverages 106
   see carbohydrates
   cholesterol and saturated fat 85, 86
   combination foods 87
   desserts 94
   dietetic foods 93
   dietitian's help with calculating
      83
   eggs 85, 112
   fat 77-78, 112-113
      calculating in diet
      hydrogenated 78
      reducing in diet 77, 111
      monounsaturated 86
      saturated 86, 100
      polysaturated 86
      trans fat   78
   fiber 97-99, 100
   flour 110
   fructose 108
   fruit 89
   glycemic index 95
   good nutrition 100
      label reading 77, 81, 86, 93, 98
   menus
      recommended 105, 106
      not recommended 103, 104
   personal preferences 84
   portion sizes 90, 114
   recipes 107, 109, 111, 117-118,
      277
   salt 96
   serving sizes 90, 114
   snacks 91
   sugar 93-95, 100
   timing of meals 91, 101
foot care 66

gestational diabetes   226
   see also pregnancy
glaucoma 166
glossary   303
glucagon 143
glucose
   use by cells 25
   high blood sugar 154
   cause of complications
   and dehydration 156
   foods to eat when ill 156
   gel for low blood sugar 141
   goals 31
   infections and 160
   ketoacidosis 156
   tablets for low blood sugar 141
glycemic index 95
glycogen
glycohemoglobin 47
glycosylated hemoglobin 47
gum disease 54
HDL see cholesterol
hemoglobin A1c 47
high blood sugar see glucose
   when sick 154-161
honeymoon phase 33
hormone 25
hydrogenated fat 78
hyperglycemia see high blood sugar
illness 154-161
impotence 172, 218
infections and high blood sugar 26-27
insulin
   chores 57
   dependent vs requiring, 38
   discovery of 17
   gestation diabetes and 227
   improvements in 21
   new 56, 232
   patient refusal 42
   pen 65

pump 61
result of none 29
receptor 189
resistance 29
types 35, 37, 56-57
insulin-dependent diabetes
    see type 1
insurance
    helping with 268
    high-risk insurance pool 267
    jobs 263
    Medical Information Bureau 265
    Medicare 266, 268
    payment for diabetes education
        266
    pump reimbursement 63
islets of Langerhans 17
jobs, getting hired   264
ketoacidosis
    causes 30, 158
    consequences of 160
    how to help   161
ketones, test 157
    see ketoacidosis
ketonuria 159
kidneys *see* complications
lactose 81
lactose free milk   81
lancets 60
laser therapy for eye disease 164-165
LDL *see* cholesterol
low blood sugar
    alcohol 138
    causes 137
    danger 39
    how to help 148
    how not to help 151
    irritability 139
    and oral meds. 68
    prevention 68
    stages of

    early 138
    more advanced 142
    advanced 143
    symptoms 139
    treatment 140, 150
magazines 319
meal plan 83
medications, side effects 170
medical identification jewelry 152
Medicare 266, 268
metabolism 25
meter *see* blood glucose meter
monounsaturated oil 86
nephropathy 48
neuropathy (nerve damage)162-163
oral medications *see* treatment
pancreas
    early research 16-19
    transplants 31
pear-shaped body type 79
periodontist 54
pharmacist 54
physician visits 51-52
    questions to ask 51
    Stands. of Medical Care 52
pills *see* treatment
    for type 1 *and* type 2   67
plate method   89
podiatrist 66
pregnancy
    type 1
        care during pregnancy 224
        large babies 224
        prevention of problems 225
    gestational 226
        diet 227
        ketone testing 227
        large babies 225
        test for 226
        who's at risk 227
    how to help 228-229

preeclampsia 225
prevention 272
protein 77
psychological issues
    see chapter 16 on feelings
pump 61
recipes
    apple coffee cake 293
    apricot vanilla "eggs" 297
    Brazilian black beans 287
    burger 286
    cabbage & white bean soup 278
    cheesecakes, fat free 292
    cheese crepes 293
    chili con carne 286
    collard greens 288
    cranberry relish 283
    dill sauce 290
    gelatin squares 297
    hot German potato salad 281
    Hungarian green beans 285
    Kung Pao Chicken 289
    pie crust 296
    potato salad, mayo 281
    pumpkin pie 294
    Renee's 2 bean salad 289
    salmon, poached 290
    strawberry sauce 294
    vanilla cream strawberry pie 295
    south of the border soup 279
    strawberry angel delight 296
    sunshine gelatin salad 282
    turkey dinner fixin's
    wild rice/mushrooms 284
research
    DCCT 47
    EDIC 48
    prevention studies 272, 274
    UKPDS 50, 69
restaurants *see dining out*
retina 166

retinopathy 48
saccharin 109
saturated fat 77, 85-87, 94, 100
school age children 234
school bus driver 237
school nurse 235
simple carbohydrate
soluble fiber *see fiber*
stress 29
stroke symptoms 170
sugar 93, 107
sugar-free 93, 109
sulfonylureas 35
supplies, carrying 65
support groups
target range   *see* exercise
teachers 235-236
teenagers 179, 239
    blood glucose goals 240
    dieting 240
    feelings 241
    life goals 241
    parents 179
    peer pressure 243
    type 2   238
temptation 181
treatment,
    decision factors
        learning problems 42
        patient resistance to 42
        patient resources 41
        physician experience 40, 46
        research findings 47
        type of diabetes 34, 56
        vision deficiency 41
        weight 41
    evaluating   52
    insulin
        intensive 57
            advantages 47
            disadvantages 49

       In young and old 49

   oral medication

      effects 68

      low blood sugar 68

      vs insulin 38

   team members 55

   type 1 vs type 2   31

type 1   11

   cause 28-29

   chores 57

   prevention

      theories 274

      research studies 274, 318

symptoms 26

   vs type 2   11

   who gets 27

type 2   11

   blood sugar testing frequency 44,
      69

   causes 29

   chores 72-73

   complications 30

   insulin 37

   prevention 272

   resistance *see* insulin

   resistance 29

   symptoms 30

   treatment *see* treatment

      vs type 1   11

   who gets 28

unsaturated fat 86

urine testing

   glucose 20, 24

      development of 20

      short-comings of 20, 21, 24

   ketone *see* ketones

   microalbuminuria 167

web sites 317-319

weight loss with Byetta 36

Here's our contact information:

For catalog and/or ordering information, please also visit our world wide website:
http://www.800books4u.com

catalog requests & retail orders:
Lincoln Publishing Incorporated
e-mail: info@800books4u.com
Tel: (503) 699-1000
Post Office Box 1499
Lake Oswego, OR 97035-0499